MW00467328

Praise

Once in a while you come across a book that stops you in your tracks and causes you to re-evaluate your lifestyle. I have just read *Informed Consent,* and that is what it did for me: I stopped and took a serious look at the choices I have made that have affected my health.

Some of us need to see the big picture, and some of us need the details. Michele has given us both in her carefully researched and sensitively written work. She has done what we haven't done or wouldn't have done for ourselves.

Mankind has been given three great powers: to think, to feel, to choose. *Informed Consent* causes us to use all three powers, and if we are wise, our choices going forward will be much more informed. We don't have control over everything in this life, but we surely should take seriously our responsibility for our health as much as we can. Michele has made that task much easier for us by writing this book.

Andrea Lyn Sims, Ph.D.
Author, *The Imposter Affect*

* * *

Michele Stanford has invested a large part of her heart in unpacking the current state of our food supply. She is passionate about bringing a health and wholeness revolution to the way we do life.

Kary Oberbrunner
Author of
ELIXIR Project
Day Job to Dream Job
The Deeper Path
and *Your Secret Name*

* * *

Eye-opening, disturbing, enlightening.

Frank Viola
Author of *From Eternity to Here*
FrankViola.org

Informed Consent

Thank you!

Michele

Informed Consent

*Critical Truths Essential to Your Health
and to the Health of Future Generations*

Michele Stanford, M.Ed., CHC

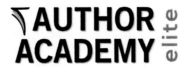

Some names and identifying details have been changed
to protect the privacy of individuals.

The information contained in this book is provided for information purposes only and it does not provide specific professional advice to any particular reader about his or her medical condition. It is in no way intended to substitute for the advice provided by your doctor or other health care professional or the labeling recommendations of any given product. You should not rely upon or follow the information contained in this book for decision making without first obtaining the advice of a physician or other health care professional. The information provided in this book is not intended to be and does not constitute health care or medical advice. Every effort has been made to make sure that the information in this book is complete and accurate. Neither the author nor the publisher shall be liable or responsible for any loss or damage incurred allegedly as a consequence of the use and application of any information or suggestions contained in this book.

Copyright @ 2017 Michele Stanford
All rights reserved
Printed in the United States of America

Published by Author Academy Elite
P.O. Box 43, Powell, OH 43035
www.AuthorAcademyElite.com

Scripture quotations taken from the New American Standard Bible® (NASB),
Copyright © 1960, 1962, 1963, 1968, 1971, 1972, 1973,
1975, 1977, 1995 by The Lockman Foundation
Used by permission. www.Lockman.org

All rights reserved. No part of this publication may be reproduced, stored in a retrieval system, or transmitted in any form or by any means – for example, electronic, photocopy, recording – without the prior written permission of the publisher. The only exception is brief quotations in printed reviews.

Paperback ISBN 978-1-64085-043-9
Hardcover ISBN 978-1-64085-044-6
Library of Congress Control Number: 2017908598

Cover design by Debbie O'Byrne
Interior design by JetLaunch, Inc.
Author photograph by Ashah Photography
Poetry retrieved from public domain

Any internet or product information printed in this book are accurate at the time of publication. They are provided as a resource with the understanding content or permanence may change. Michele Stanford or the publisher do not vouch for their content or permanence.

In memory of my daddy–

You were the most Christ-like man I have ever known.
You were no theologian, nor were you one to discuss doctrine.
Rather, you quietly lived out what you believed,
day in and day out,
filled with the Fruit of the Spirit:
love, joy, peace, patience, kindness,
goodness, faithfulness, gentleness,
and self-control – every day – to all those
with whom you interacted.
Thank you for your example, for your support,
and for your unconditional love.
I love you to the moon and back!
I miss you every day.
I am forever your *D.B.*!

Contents

Foreword xi
Acknowledgements xiii
Note to Reader xv
Introduction 1

Part I—The Red Pill

1: Flashback 11
2: The State of our Food Address 23
3: They Did *What* to My Food?! 34
4: What's for Dinner? 65
5: Remember Nuremberg? 81
6: Toxic Overload 112

Part II—Hope and Healing

7: The Hope-Filled Journey 123
8: Wellness: An Act of Worship 125
9: Real Food is Real Good 128
10: Tools for Your Toolbox 155
11: What's Life Got to Do With It? 176
12: You've Got Wings, Baby! 186
Appendix A 191
Appendix B 193
Appendix C 197
Resources 201
Endnotes 205
About the Author 219

Foreword

As a person who has been studying health and wellness for over 20 years, I thought I had a great grasp on how we have evolved into such a sick society. After reading Michele's book I have to admit that the attention is in the details…and she provides plenty of them that I have either forgotten over the years or missed entirely. Also many things that I had overcomplicated she has delivered in an easy to understand, entertaining, and informative book.

This book is for the person who is just dipping their toe into the water of what it means to eat and live in a more sustainable and healthy way, as well as the seasoned pioneer in the wellness space. It contains something unique for everyone, no matter the length of their journey or struggle.

The best piece of the book in my opinion is that Michele shares her story, her fears, and her health accomplishments, which tell us we are all more alike than we think. She is not alone in her concerns for her health and she sheds light on why we should all be MORE concerned about what is happening to our world today. I am thrilled that she is bringing these topics to light and I consider this book a true gift for those who have YET to discover what their future holds due to the choices they are making right this minute.

This book will open your eyes, it will inform you, it will challenge your thinking and most of all, I am sure it will inspire *some* change in you no matter how big or small. No one is too advanced in their health knowledge to not glean a bit of truth from this book.

Well done 110% Michele!

Carmen Hunter
Founder, The Institute For Functional Health Coaching™
Certified Health Coach and seeker of health for all people

Acknowledgements

Ross and Trevor, my cup overflows. Your very existence is the most precious gift I possess. It is an honor to be your mom. Thank you for your willingness to share a tiny piece of our story. I love you both immeasurably; truly my cup runneth over.

Mom, thank you for your support during this process and for your grace during the difficult times; it means the world to me. I love you.

Monica, my life is blessed and enriched through your friendship. Your support and encouragement these many years are beyond measure. Thank you for always being there for me and for standing with me during the hard times. Jesus sent you to hold me up when the pain was unspeakably unbearable and I could not stand; you kept me from falling and for that I will be eternally grateful. Much love to you, friend.

Kary Oberbrunner, my coach and mentor, this would not have been possible without your support, encouragement, and example. Your belief in me is a gift not soon forgotten. Thank you.

A special thank you to my dear friends and team members in ministry at Courageously Free Women: Vicki Kloosterhouse, Ann Brainard, Jeanne Schmidt, Elle Roetzel, Niccie Kleigl, Teresea Alesch, and Sabrina Alley. Your support, encouragement, and prayers carried me through. Thank you, sweet friends. It is an honor to serve alongside each of you.

Jim Akers, you challenge me and inspire me. Thank you for your impact on my life.

There are many friends who encouraged and supported me who deserve a very big thank you: Linda Marie Zupanic, for all the long talks when we were both in a precarious place; Joel Kessel, for affirming that this message needs to be shared; Jeff Glass, Terry Stafford, Cathy Yost, for your encouragement and support; small acts of kindness have tremendous impact.

A special thank you to Andrea and to Laura for your feedback and kind words; it was invaluable. To Carmen, thank you for *all* that you do. I am grateful every day that our paths crossed.

A very special thank you to Ann* for your friendship. Your selfless act of kindness that infamous night and your friendship through the years have been blessings for which I am forever grateful.

To those whose works I have cited here and to many others who are dedicated to speaking truth. My life is different because of it and for that I thank you!

Finally, I want to thank all of those farmers who are committed to organic and sustainable practices and who are dedicated to providing their local communities with healthful, nourishing foods; without you, food freedom would not be possible. Thank you!

Note to Reader

The information contained here can be complex and at times technical. However, I have striven to make this information accessible to everyone, regardless of education level.

Entire books and volumes of books have been written on the varying subjects here, so this is by necessity not an extensive discussion on these topics; rather I have extrapolated the most relevant and pertinent information so that you can make informed decisions about your health and that of your family. As well, I have provided Appendices and Resource pages so that you may continue to educate yourself on these topics.

As a Christian, this book is underpinned by the tenets of my faith. If you are of another faith, this book is still for you. Know that you are loved and the information contained here is for you and your family, also. It is important for all of humanity.

Introduction

I didn't say it would be easy, Neo.
I just said it would be the truth.
Morpheus, *The Matrix*

Forgetting pain is convenient. Remembering it, agonizing.
But recovering the truth is worth the suffering.
The Cheshire Cat, *Alice in Wonderland*

Twenty-three years ago I lay in the emergency room all alone and I was told that I had to have surgery, immediately, or I could die. At home was my then-husband, my almost three year old son, and my nine month old son who was sick with walking pneumonia and asthma, requiring breathing treatments via a nebulizer every four hours. The problem with that was my then-husband was an absentee husband who was in denial that our youngest son was very sick, and who had absolutely no idea what medications to use or how to give him treatments.

I was alone. I had driven myself to the hospital because my then-husband would not allow me to call a friend to drive me or to stay with the children while he drove me; that would be an imposition. Two days earlier we had just purchased a new car for me and I was not allowed to drive it to the hospital 30 miles away in the event I had some sort of attack and wrecked the new car; so instead, in excruciating pain I had to drive the old clunker work truck to the hospital. Such were the makings of my life.

| 1 |

I wanted desperately to go home, make arrangements for the children, and return the next morning for surgery. *Well, you can go home if you want*, exclaimed the doctor, his voice dripping more with sarcasm than compassion, *but there is no guarantee you will live through the night. Your appendix is extremely inflamed; I'm surprised it has not already ruptured, and there is a very real possibility that it will burst and you will hemorrhage to death before you can make it back to the hospital. But it's up to you.*

Terrified does not begin to describe my reaction at that point. Faced with possibility of death. Alone. Very sick baby at home. Panicked. Mind racing. I need to call someone. Anyone. Tell *somebody* I might die tonight… And who is going to take care of my baby…?! No one who knows how to take care of him and knows what he needs. That, more than dying, was my greatest fear. Absolute horror. It was one of the worst experiences of my life. I can still see the doctor in his white lab coat towering over me as I lie on the cold, steel table in the blindingly bright light in that frigidly cold room. Freezing. Excruciating physical pain. Now terrified. The starkness of the room mirrored the stark truth of that moment.

I was allowed to walk out to the nurses' station and make a few phone calls (this was back in the day before cell phones, except for the big clunky kind in a big box): one to my then-husband, and one to friend and work colleague, Ann. My friend told me that she and her husband, Jay, would be there as soon as possible. Slight relief. At least someone would be there to receive the news if I didn't make it. So we waited… and waited… still no Ann. As I was being rolled down the hallway, approaching those dubious double doors, the entrance to oblivion, Ann and Jay burst on the scene, breathless. *I'm sorry it took us so long, but Washington Road was a nightmare to navigate!*

Yes, you see, it was Sunday evening of Master's Week in Augusta; a drive that should have taken 20 minutes, took over an hour. But finally, someone to hold my purse and move the old clunker that was in jeopardy of being towed from the two-hour parking at the emergency room and someone to just be there waiting to make sure I made it! She kissed my forehead, told me she loved me, and that they would be there when I came out.

We are still friends, Ann and me. I am forever grateful to Jay and to her for their friendship and their love, especially that night. And yes, they were in my room waiting for me. Jay had moved the clunker work truck... *If you look out the window, you can see the truck; it is at 11:00.* Forever grateful.

The next morning the surgeon came in with a surprising announcement. *The surgery went well. It was a pleasure operating on someone thin for a change; nice and clean because I didn't have to cut through a lot of fat.* Hmm. Okay. *You have an infection in the portion of your small intestine that attaches to the appendix. If you had been prepped for a bowel operation, I would have taken that portion out.* Excuse me! WHAT?!

One thing I know: the Lord protected me that night; He did not allow that "doctor" to butcher my body.

A gastroenterologist was called in, Dr. Jones. He was an older gentleman with a pleasing bedside manner, kind, and compassionate. In fact, he was what some might call 'old school' even then. He spent an hour with me that day, questioning me about my life, probing for specific details; details I did not particularly want to share because they were not all pretty. I was in an emotionally, verbally, and at times physically, abusive marriage to an adulterous alcoholic. I had a sick baby and a three year old, both of whom I was primarily raising on my own. I was working as a legal assistant. I had virtually no support system since our families lived out of state. And that's the short list. Life was hard and I was struggling... alone.

Six weeks later I underwent several tests to determine if I had Crohn's disease. Thankfully, I did not. Dr. Jones determined that the infection in my intestine had been caused by chronic, severe stress. *You must learn to manage your stress.* I made a joke and laughed. He did not. Rather sternly rebuked me. *This is serious. You must find a way to manage your stress.*

Thus began my twenty plus years struggle to manage my digestive issues.

And manage was all I could manage.

In the beginning, there were times when I would get the same symptoms I had experienced in the week leading up to my surgery. It was during those times that Dr. Jones advised me to go on a "soft food" diet (He was on the cusp of what I needed to heal, but not quite there. I will explain this in Part II). He would call me periodically, over the years, to check on me. At one point he wanted to run more tests. Even as he suggested testing, he admitted that he did not believe I suffered with any of the conditions for which I would be tested, but it was necessary to rule out those conditions. He admitted that he really had no idea what was wrong with me. He admitted that the eventual outcome might be either surgery or prescription medication, neither of which I considered a viable option. I did not have insurance at the time, so testing was out of the question. In hindsight, I realize having no insurance was a blessing in disguise. Had I gone forward with testing, I now know that my problems would have been made worse. So I did what I could to manage my symptoms…for twenty years. Twenty. Years.

Fast forward ten years, I was a divorced, single mother of teen and pre-teen boys. *Oy vey!* I was diagnosed with hypothyroidism and I was in very early perimenopause. My general practitioner, who was also my friend and fellow choir member at church, was incredulous when I told her that I was in perimenopause. *That's just not possible. You are too young.* Blood tests don't lie. She was stunned. She understood the hypothyroidism, but not early perimenopause. Thyroid medication prescription. Check. *You will need to take this every day for the rest of your life or you could die.* (A very common health issue; but should it be?) What no one told me, and what I later learned through research, was that my endocrine system was completely out of balance and it was directly related to my gut issues and the unrelenting stress I was under; there were, and had been, some very dark years where I had been under persistent, chronic stress.

Fast forward another ten years and I am back "home" to be near my parents who are aging and both of whom are dealing with serious health issues of cancer, heart disease, kidney disease caused by chemotherapy, the recurrence of cancer and the subsequent further chemotherapy treatments, severe sickness as a result, *ad nausem*. Continual roller coaster ride courtesy of allopathic medicine.

At the time I was teaching and because of the health conditions of my parents – no immune system to speak of – my mother asked me to get a flu shot so that I would not bring any illnesses from school to their home. I resisted, but eventually I acquiesced and immediately became ill. For six months I suffered from extreme fatigue and other symptoms. It was all I could do just to get through each day. I thought perhaps my thyroid medication needed to be adjusted, so I went to my new general practitioner who told me that no, my levels looked fine, but for good measure, here is another prescription for a higher dose anyway. Along with the extreme fatigue, I began suffering from symptoms of atrial fibrillation, interestingly, at about the same times every day, give or take an hour. The symptoms would come on so suddenly I would need to clutch my lectern to remain standing while gasping for air in the middle of a discussion of John Donne's sonnet "Batter My Heart" trying to maintain control, appear normal so as not to alarm my students. My heart certainly felt as if it were being battered!

Six months into this I decided that there was something very wrong with me and that it was more than just the digestive issues I was continuing to (barely) manage. It was time to find answers on my own, so I spent every spare moment researching, starting with my gut issues. I happened upon an article which dealt with adverse reactions to the flu shot. As I read down the list... check... check... check... and it was then that I began to connect the dots. Six months later, one year after the flu shot, I returned to my general practitioner for my annual check-up and thyroid testing. Not surprisingly, my thyroid results were off the chart because I was on a higher dose than was necessary, hence the atrial fibrillation symptoms (again, the Lord was protecting me), so he put me on a much lower dose than I had previously been taking; rather than put me back on the original dosage, he lowered my dosage to the point my symptoms of fatigue became worse because I was not getting enough thyroid medication. *Sigh.*

The fatigue caused by the flu shot combined with the fatigue from insufficient thyroid medication rendered getting through each day a feat the size of climbing Mount Everest. At this appointment, I mentioned that the flu shot had made me sick and caused a number of symptoms. *The flu shot cannot make you sick.* Well, it did and I explained my findings to him. *The flu shot CANNOT make you sick!* He was getting angry. I also told him that I had used therapeutic grade essential oils to successfully support my body's immune function in regards to an infection that I had. *Essential oils do not work.* Yes, actually, they did. It was at this point he stood up, walked to the door, and said, *I refuse to treat anyone who believes the things you do!* then turned and stormed out. Yes, you read that correctly. Good riddance. Best thing an allopathic doctor ever did for me!

I began to see a Naturopathic Doctor (ND) who had me complete an in depth health history beginning with my mother's pregnancy with me, then ran a battery of tests. It was determined that I was suffering from HPA-Axis dysfunction and Hashimoto's thyroiditis, an autoimmune disorder where the immune system attacks the thyroid. In other words, my body was attacking itself; but I had hope now. The beauty of naturopathic doctors and functional medicine doctors is that they look to the root cause of an issue rather than slapping a band-aide on symptoms. They treat the body as a whole system, rather than compartmentalized; and not just the body, but the mind and emotions also. It is all inextricably linked. With the assistance of my ND and the knowledge I was gaining through my own research, I was equipped with what I needed to begin the journey to healing, not only my thyroid and my HPA Axis dysfunction, but my digestive issues as well.

Am I healed today? Not completely. Twenty years of disease cannot be healed overnight, especially when dealing with gut issues and the problems of scarring in my intestines from that initial infection, the autoimmunity, and the endocrine imbalances. It takes time. I also had a setback last year after an acute exposure to mold. If only it were so simple; but our bodies are exposed to a plethora of toxins each day, pathogens invade, many different organs and mechanisms are involved. Detoxification is an ongoing process. It takes time. It is a process.

I am on the road to healing and I am so much better now after having applied the information which I am sharing with you. I am healing! For the first time in twenty plus years, I am making progress! I share this so you will understand that there is no magic bullet or 10-day miracle cure; but there is real, lasting change and improvement. Our Creator designed our bodies with a beautiful, innate ability to heal itself when given the right substances.

You see, dear reader, this book isn't about me. My purpose in writing is to share all that I have learned, so that you, too, can begin a journey on the road to healing. To be sure, others have written entire books on the varying subjects contained here. I have read many of them and I reference them. I have spent hours and hours researching online databases such as PubMed and others credible sources. My desire is to distill the most important, the most pertinent information into one resource so that you can begin your own journey without having to spend months and years researching as I have done.

I must warn you, though, there are many truths contained in this book that you may find unpalatable and shocking; in fact, you may be quite skeptical. The truth is not always easy.

Another thing I know: Once you know truth, you can't unknow it. Once you know truth, you have a moral obligation and a moral imperative to apply and to share that truth; there is a responsibility associated with it.

This message is profoundly important and it must not be ignored. You must know these truths if you want to regain your health, ensure the health of our children, and the health of future generations. I learned this information too late to help my daddy; the damage done him through allopathic medicine was too great.

It is not too late for you!

Therefore, I urge you, brethren, by the mercies of God, to present your bodies a living sacrifice, acceptable to God, which is your spiritual service of worship, And do not be conformed to this world, but be transformed by the renewing of your mind, so that you may prove what the will of God is, that which is good and acceptable and perfect. Romans 12:1-2

Michele Stanford

Part I
The Red Pill

This is your last chance [Neo]. After this, there is no
turning back. You take the blue pill - the story ends,
you wake up in your bed and believe whatever you want
to believe. You take the red pill - you stay in Wonderland
and I show you how deep the rabbit-hole goes.
Morpheus, *The Matrix*

1 | Flashback

The human body heals itself and nutrition provides the resources to accomplish the task.
Roger Williams, Ph.D.

Medicine is far from having decreased human sufferings as much as it endeavors to make us believe. Indeed, the number of deaths from infectious diseases has greatly diminished. But we still must die in a much larger proportion from degenerative diseases.
Dr. Alexis Carrell in "Man, the Unknown"

How have we become a people, a society that is so apathetic, so complacent? May I also suggest, complicit?

Remember this question; keep it in the back of your mind. I will come back to it and provide an answer in the next and following chapters; but first, I am going to ask for a little latitude. You see, you've come into this story in the middle and so to understand where we are, we need to understand how we got here and how things once were. In literature, when a story goes from the present to the past, it's referred to as a flashback. We are going to take a journey into the not too distant past. Indulge me as I take you into my classroom for a lesson in poetry and a lesson in history.

* * *

First, I want to introduce you to a poem that is just as relevant today as when it was written in 1902 at the height of the Industrial Revolution. This is one of the poems I taught in my poetry unit each year. At the end of the unit, students were required to choose a poem to recite and to craft a detailed explication. Most of the males *always* chose this poem. Every year. They think the poem is simple and easy, but, in fact, it is full of imagery that stirs all of the five senses, and includes some kinesthetic imagery as well. Don't worry; no detailed poetry explanation here, just a little summary and a little imagery to keep in mind as we explore and begin to understand why we are a nation of sick people. I want you to keep these images in mind throughout this book.

This poem is rich with meaning. Have some fun with it. Poetry was originally an oral tradition; it was recited aloud, not silently read to oneself. It was almost always accompanied by music. Stand up. Read it out loud! I promise, it will bring an entirely different perspective.

Cargoes (1902)
by: John Masefield

Quinquereme* of Nineveh from distant Ophir,
Rowing home to haven in sunny Palestine,
With a cargo of ivory,
And apes and peacocks,
Sandalwood, cedarwood, and sweet white wine.

Stately Spanish galleon coming from the Isthmus,
Dipping through the Tropics by the palm-green shores,
With a cargo of diamonds,
Emeralds, amethysts,
Topazes, and cinnamon, and gold moidores.

---

*   A quinquereme was an ancient ship

Dirty British coaster with a salt-caked smoke-stack,
Butting through the Channel in the mad March days,
With a cargo of Tyne coal,
Road-rails, pig-lead,
Firewood, iron-ware, and cheap tin trays.

In the first stanza, you see a galley on its way home to ancient Palestine from Ophir, believed to be an ancient city in Africa. It is referenced in the Bible as being a place from where gold was brought to King Solomon for use in the building of the Temple. The cargo it is carrying is exotic: ivory, apes, peacocks, certainly not things you would find in Palestine. The heady aroma of sandalwood, cedarwood, and sweet white wine filled the air and overwhelmed the senses. The oarsmen were rowing, which speaks to a gentle, leisurely journey. Uninhibited. Peaceful. Serene.

In the second stanza, you see a Spanish galleon. It is the period of New World exploration in the tropical Caribbean. The cargo this galleon is carrying exudes wealth for it is filled with the sparkle of gemstones reflecting the light, the pungent scent of the rare and expensive spice, cinnamon, and the twinkle of gold coins in the blazing sun. Here, too, the oars are dipping in the water, very little sound from this ship commissioned by the Spanish government, proudly bringing home its spoils. Warm tropical breezes usher the crew on to Spain.

By the third stanza you see that industrialization has arrived. There are no oarsmen. This coaster is powered by coal. Pollution. The smoke-stack is coated with salt from the English Channel as the ocean air is stirred by the storms of early spring and the waves batter this vessel. Its cargo is the end result of industrialized products. Dirty. Smelly. Noisy. Items that pollute the earth and assault the faculties. Poisonous.

Masefield was making a statement with this poem as so many poets and writers have done. He was speaking out against the blight he observed. Masefield romanticized previous eras in history, which to be sure had their share of problems. The quinquereme oarsmen were most certainly slaves; the wealthy cargo of the Spanish galleon was stolen by conquest – not exactly ideal societies. However, he wanted to make a point about the perhaps unintended and unforeseen results of industrialization. He did not like what he was witnessing as the Industrial Revolution roared forward; rather he was longing for simpler times; cleaner times. Imagine, pristine air suddenly becomes chocked with smoke and grim. New, never before felt, seen, or whiffed odiferous plumbs hanging in the air. Shocking. Unwelcome.

Charles Dickens at the beginning of the Industrial Revolution used his novels to make statements about the new age of industrialized agriculture with the advent of slaughter houses, which he found abhorrent, to horrendous working conditions, and everything in between. He was very vocal on his dislike of the significant changes taking place in the world and their impact on society, which he viewed as negative rather than positive.

As well, this was the "Age of Enlightenment" meaning science was the new ideology and Darwin's *Origin of the Species* had burst on the scene and rocked everyone's world. Matthew Arnold wrote "Dover Beach" to lament the loss of Christian faith as a result of Darwin's theories. It was a time when science ruled and faith (and logic) walked away.

Why did we not listen?

On the one hand, much has changed in the last one hundred years; good and positive changes. On the other hand, some things have not changed in the last one hundred years; rather they have continued to poison the population. Industrialization is alive and well and disordering lives. Don't get me wrong, I'm all for modernization; I rather like my indoor plumbing. However, there are some things that should not be altered, modernized, or created in an industrial setting. There are laws of nature that should be respected, God's laws; to not respect nature's laws leads to catastrophic consequences. Masefield and Dickens understood this; Arnold understood this.

* * *

Life in all its fullness is Mother Nature obeyed.
Weston A. Price, DDS

The Work of Weston A. Price, DDS

Dr. Price, originally from Ontario, moved to Cleveland, Ohio, to open his dental practice in the early 20th Century. He was not only a dentist, but he was also a scientist and a humanitarian. He spent many years studying the rise in dental caries and the causes, using scientific methods and research, as well as clinical observation. He postulated that the rise in tooth decay was due to the malnutrition of individuals, concluding that perhaps the cause was a result of some missing necessary ingredients in the diet. He decided that in order to prove this theory, he needed a control group of people who were isolated from industrialized society. Thus began a several-years-long journey to remote places around the globe.

Dr. Price visited remote villages in Switzerland; islands off the coast of Scotland; Eskimos in Alaska; Native American Indian tribes; islands in the South Sea; tribes of Peru and the Amazon Basin; African tribes; Aboriginals in Australia; and isolated tribes in New Zealand. All of the groups of peoples he visited were completely isolated from industrialized society and lived entirely on indigenous foods. However, he had one modern invention that he used: the camera, with which he recorded the stellar health and vitality of these people groups as well as document the decline in health when these groups were exposed to industrialized foods.

In 1939, Dr. Price, because he wanted to make his findings known and accessible to all people, including the lay person, chronicled his journey, findings, and data, including photographs, in his opus, *Nutrition and Physical Degeneration*.[1] It is a tome, but it is truly fascinating reading! It is to be noted here that he paid for all of his travel, research, and publishing with monies he earned from his dental practice. He rejected offers from companies to fund his efforts so that his work would reflect the truth he was seeking, unbiased and without interference.

What Dr. Price discovered is quite astounding and profoundly pertinent, important, and relevant for us today, perhaps more so than ever before.

Nutrient Dense Foods

Dr. Price very quickly was able to determine that the rise in tooth decay was, in fact, directly related to industrial, modernized foods. What he found completely astounding was that with the introduction of modernized foods, within one generation, the people groups began experiencing not only dental caries and dental deformities, but also degenerative diseases. Within ONE generation! Additionally, he observed that the increase in disease was rapid and increased in severity with each successive generation and it was very much like what he was witnessing in American and European modern societies.

Dr. Price observed that these isolated people groups possessed strong immunity to disease as well as no malformation. He noticed that these peoples would use certain foods which were often hard to acquire, but which provided certain elements such as iron, manganese, iodine, and copper. They knew, intuitively, that they needed these foods. Additionally, all of these groups, no matter where in the world they were located, ate foods that were very nutrient dense and all groups ate meat and/or fish, less often the muscle meats, but always the organs, and they used the bones, and just about every part of the animal. Some groups ate primarily raw foods, including raw meat. Some groups ate primarily cooked foods; but, they all ate foods that were highly nutrient dense.

Another interesting tidbit is that these groups would keep in their knapsacks a ball of clay and they would use a small piece to make an infusion into which they would dip their food. The clay attracts pathogens and carries them out of the body and prevents "sour stomach." It is now popular to consume such clay in order to detox from heavy metals. As you will see, we have a lot to learn from these groups of people.

Dr. Price noted that none of these people groups lived exclusively on plant food; they all included meat in some form in their diet. Depending on the region in which they lived, the meat of choice varied. Those living near the ocean and rivers, consumed large amounts of fish and fish eggs. The Eskimos consumed large amounts of fish, but also the blubber, which is rich in fat. It should be mentioned that these groups ate foods indigenous to the region in which they lived and all of these groups consumed foods that were highly nutritious.

Dr. Price described these people groups as having "excellent bodies" and free of any deformities or degenerative diseases. He describes them as having no tooth decay and no need for glasses. They were adept at supporting their nutrition with foods which offered protection from disease and which promoted vitality and robust health; he observed that they kept these secret just as modern societies keep secret weapons of warfare.

All of the groups also ate grains, which were properly prepared, and definitely not refined. We will discuss later in Chapter 9 the methods of proper, traditional preparation of grains. Dr. Price, being the scientist, analyzed everything. He tested the chemical compositions of the foods, tracing the amount of minerals and vitamins each contained; he tested different grains, and different preparation methods, and experimented using these different grains and preparations on rats. The rats fed properly prepared whole grains thrived; the rats fed refined white flour did not and they were riddled with tooth decay, degenerative disease, and did not reproduce. The third group was underweight. His researched confirmed what he was witnessing in these people groups: Properly prepared grains were an important part of what Dr. Price called the building blocks to robust health, grains being only one of many other important and necessary foods which include fat-soluble vitamins A, D, and what he referred to as "Activator X" which we now believe to be Vitamin K_2, that can only be absorbed in conjunction with the consumption of animal fats.

There is a reason why your grandmother slathered those greens with butter! I will discuss these principles in more detail in Part II; for now, understand Dr. Price observed that animal fats, protein, properly prepared carbohydrates, and unrefined foods, were all necessary components of a diet that led to vibrant health.

Preparing the Next Generation

In an interesting observation, Dr. Price documented that in each of the people groups there were times of special feeding for women prior to conception, and indeed prior to marriage; often in the six months leading up to marriage, girls were given special diets significantly high in nutrition to prepare their bodies for conception. This was observed in every group he studied. In some groups, the males were also given special diets. According to Dr. Price, the process of degeneration is not something that happens after birth, but rather before conception. He noted that "germal blight" was (and is) the cause of degeneration. As I stated earlier, within one generation of incorporating processed foods into the diet, degeneration was noted.

Dr. Price cited an article written by Dr. J.C. Drummond for the *Journal of the American Medical Association*[2] in 1938, wherein he discussed the decline in fertility rates and Dr. Drummond drew a direct correlation between the decrease in fertility and the advent of milled and processed flour which made it accessible to the masses. In other words, diet, specifically a processed foods diet, played a major role in the decrease of fertility rates. I posit that this is still the case today. The incidences of infertility have continued to rise; there are more and more fertility clinics all over the world, something that was unheard of 100 years ago.

Another interesting observation regards infants; in many of the people groups, after birth the infant was wrapped in an absorbent moss, which was changed daily. The infants were not washed; rather the oily film covering the baby was left intact. Modern society will find this practice deplorable, but in 1931 Multanomah County Hospital in Portland, Oregon adopted this practice (not washing the infant) and left the film intact and only washed the babies' bottoms. What they found was that the incidence of skin rashes completely disappeared and the film naturally disappeared over time. Nature provides everything needed!

As I stated earlier, Dr. Price noticed that physical changes occurred within one generation. The same is also true of a return to a diet of real food. Dr. Price relates many such stories of a return to robust health after adopting a diet of real food with plenty of animal products, animal fats, and vegetables rich in minerals and vitamins. Not only is it possible within one generation, but it is also possible within *a* generation. Dr. Price illustrated this concept by examining a mother and her two daughters.

With the first daughter, the mother was in labor 53 hours and she was quite invalid for many months after giving birth. The child had a deformation of the dental arches, she was a very nervous and anxious child, and she had begun to stoop at the age of ten. Prior to conception, the mother's nutrition was based primarily on a modernized diet, full of refined and processed foods. By the time of conception of the second daughter 4 years later, the mother had adopted a nutritious diet free of processed and refined foods. She was in labor only 3 hours and she was back to her normal activities very quickly following birth. The second daughter had normal dental arches, without any deformities, and exhibited strong, robust health, without the nervous and anxious tendencies of her older sister.

Dr. Price related this story to make the point that physical and mental disabilities are rarely genetic in the way we think of these things as being inherited, but rather the result of nutritional deficiencies that inhibit normal development. The health of *both* parents *prior* to conception are vital for the health of each successive generation. In fact, a recent study[3] links the health of the father and his eating habits prior to conception to deficiencies in his children. Another study[4] demonstrates a direct correlation between the eating of junk food by the parents to metabolic disorders in their children. Over 75 years after Dr. Price noted these same findings, the modern world is finally catching up; in fact, these studies do not mention the research of Dr. Price. Why has it taken so long for modernized society to acknowledge the work of Dr. Price, albeit unwittingly? The answer to this question lies in the pages ahead.

Soil Fertility

An entire chapter in Dr. Price's book is dedicated to soil depletion and the impact that it has on animals and plant life. He observed that the people groups went to great lengths to conserve and preserve the integrity of the soil. He noticed that animals fed rapidly growing grasses thrived, their milk supply was greater, and the mortality rate of their calves was significantly less than those cows fed grains. This would seem to be common sense, but what Dr. Price also noticed was that in areas of the United States where agriculture was "industrialized" the mortality rates were higher. Per Dr. Price, the minerals of the soil were being carted off to the big cities, rather than being used to replenish the soil. If the soil is depleted of minerals, the plants and the animals suffer and thus the people suffer. Most of the produce in the grocery stores today is deficient in the minerals that would be present were proper farming practices in place, but which are difficult to maintain on large scale operations.

Consequently, even if you are eating fresh produce, unless it is organic, and sometimes not even then, that produce is deficient in the nutrients that your body needs. Many modern diseases are the result of the absence of vital minerals and vitamins found in food; but if the food supply is also deficient in these important elements, then we are hard pressed to get them in adequate quantities in our diets. While supplements may help, the majority of supplements are synthetic and not assimilated by our bodies; in other words, you are literally throwing money down the toilet.

Dr. Price lamented, "The complacency with which the masses of the people as well as the politicians view our trend is not unlike the drifting of a merry party in the rapids above a great cataract. There seems to be no appropriate sense of impending doom."[5] And he was correct; for years there has not been a sense of doom to what we are doing to our food and the precious soil in which we grow our food. However, the tide is finally shifting and there is a growing awareness of the deficiencies as well as the dangers present in our food supply.

Effect on Society

I want to make one final point about the work of Dr. Price. As he studied America, he noticed that not only was physical degeneration rampant, but so was the incidence of mental disturbances, lowered IQ, and the rise of delinquent behavior, all of which he attributed to nutritional deficiencies. Price observed:

> After one has lived among the primitive racial stock in different parts of the world and studied them in their isolation, few impressions can be more vivid than that of the absence of prisons and asylums. Few, if any, of the problems which confront modern civilization are more serious and disturbing than the progressive increase in the percentage of individuals with unsocial traits and a lack of responsibility.[6]

Dr. Price wrote those words in 1938. Read them again. Let them sink in.

How much more relevant are those words today?

At the same time Dr. Price was making these observations during the 1930s and leading up to the rise of the Nazi party and World War II, Hitler and his cronies were systematically trying to eliminate these very types of individuals from the human race and/or experimenting on them (more on this subject in Chapter 5). It was common belief that those individuals with some form of mental or physical disability should be segregated from society and sterilized so as not to pass on the deformity or disability (which Dr. Price has shown to be a result of a modernized diet full of refined and processed foods). The very society and societal changes that caused these maladies in individuals was the very society demonizing the victims and seeking to eliminate them. The atrocities perpetrated on these individuals (and others), as you know, were horrific.

These atrocities are still being perpetrated today.

2

The State of our Food Address

Do not participate in the unfruitful deeds of darkness,
but instead even expose them; for it is disgraceful even
to speak of the things which are done by them in secret.
But all things become visible when they are exposed
by the light, for everything that becomes visible is light.
For this reason it says, Awake, sleeper,
And arise from the dead, and Christ will shine on you.
Ephesians 5:11-14

Just as there are predatory birds, there are predatory ideas.
Elie Wiesel

So, what is the big deal about industrialized and heavily refined foods? Well, they're industrialized and heavily refined. They are no longer a whole food; in fact, most refined "food" is not really food at all, rather a concoction of chemicals assembled together that are made to look and taste like food. They are food-like products and not real food at all. Let's examine one, a favorite snack for many, especially children.

Cheez-Its. Who doesn't like Cheez-Its? I used to love them. Just ask my students. They were my go to comfort food, salty, crunchy, cheesy; but after I made the switch to real, whole food, they no longer tasted, well, like food. They tasted more like cardboard. Back in the day when life was dark and bleak, I always had a box in my desk at work. Work was my happy place, the place where I felt safe and comfortable and accepted. That's how they became my comfort food. I associated them with a safe and comfortable space. Let's examine the ingredients:

> Enriched flour (wheat flour, niacin, reduced iron, thiamine mononitrate [Vitamin B1], riboflavin [Vitamin B2], folic acid). Vegetable oil (soybean and palm oil with TBHQ for freshness). Cheese made with skim milk (skim milk, whey protein, cheese cultures, salt, enzymes, annatto extract for color). Contains 2% or less of salt, paprika, yeast, paprika oleoresin for color, soy lecithin).

First up, enriched flour. Sounds nutritious, right? You decide. As you know, flour is made from ground whole wheat (or wheat berry) and it has three layers: the bran, the germ, and the endosperm. In order to make white flour, the bran is removed which contains fiber, protein, and trace minerals. The germ is also removed which contains B vitamins and trace minerals as well as some fats, which is also removed to extend the shelf life. What's left is the endosperm which is ground into flour and is yellowish in color. It is then bleached with chlorine or benzoyl peroxide to oxidize the flour which gives it the white color. This process not only leaves behind chemical residue, it also destroys any nutrients that must be added back in the form of synthetic vitamins and minerals; these make up the next several items on the ingredients list: niacin, reduced iron, thiamin mononitrate (vitamin B1) riboflavin (vitamin B12), and folic acid.

These synthetic vitamins are molecularly different than those found in nature, and they are therefore, not recognized by the body which means they are not bioavailable. Additionally, with the removal of the bran and the germ, the "flour" is broken down more quickly in the body which raises blood sugar levels. When the liver can't metabolize the overload of blood sugar, the remainder is stored as fat. While "enriched" flour may *sound* healthy, it is anything but healthy. Most processed foods contain enriched flour and the white flour you buy by the five-pound bag is the same flour. And if that were not enough, this wheat is chemically modified and doused with herbicides immediately before harvest, which I will discuss in detail in the next chapter.

The next ingredient after enriched flour and the added synthetic vitamins is vegetable oil (soybean and palm oil with TBHQ for freshness). The first problem is that soybeans are genetically modified and the palm oil industry is linked to human rights violations, including child labor, and the palm fruit is not sustainably grown and harvested.[7] The TBHQ is the abbreviation for "tertiary butyl hydroquinone," a form of butane, a/k/a, lighter fluid. It is a chemical preservative originally developed for use with petroleum and rubber products. The FDA allows 0.02% of the total oil to contain TBHQ. This just begs the question: If it is safe to eat, then why does there need to be a limit on how much can be placed in your food? And if you are eating a lot of refined, packaged foods, are you getting more than the 0.02%? High doses of TBHQ (1-4 grams) can cause a multitude of physical problems including nausea, vomiting, delirium, hyperactivity, asthma, dermatitis, especially in children, and can cause estrogen disruption in women, to name a few. The "for freshness" is not sounding so fresh after all. Stay away from open flames while you munch on your crackers!

The process involved in creating soybean oil is one I hope you find deplorable. This is the same process for corn oil and canola oil that line the shelves of the supermarket. The label "vegetable" oil is somewhat misleading; it is actually a seed oil. You can't press a soybean seed, cottonseed, or a grain of corn and get oil. It must be extracted using high temperatures and the application of hexane, which is a solvent made from crude oil. The Centers for Disease Control and Prevention classifies hexane as a neurotoxin and the Environmental Protection Agency considers it a hazardous air pollutant and continually monitors its release into the environment. Once the oil is released from the seed by the use of the toxic solvent, hexane, it is a dark, thick, smelly gunk.

The use of bleach is then applied to this smelly gunk to clean the color and deodorize the smell. This process is called degunking. Not only are free radicals produced, but these solvents and chemicals leave their residue. This same process is used to create the white lard-type product from cottonseed, which isn't an edible plant, but is considered a vegetable in the world of botany because its plant fibers are similar to those of edible plants; hemp, jute, and flax also fall under this classification.

Cheese made with skim milk (skim milk, why protein, cheese cultures, salt, enzymes, annatto extract) is next up on our list. In Chapter 4, I will show you what goes on in a Concentrated Animal Feeding Operation (CAFO), which includes the beef, dairy, pork, and poultry industries, so for now, just know that these animal products contain hormones and antibiotics and live in horrendous conditions. Skim milk, pasteurized and denatured, obviously has had all of the fat, or cream removed, with Vitamins A and D added back in which are naturally occurring in grass-fed cows and which are fat soluble, meaning the fat is needed in order for our bodies to absorb those vitamins. Adding synthetic Vitamins A and D is futile; they are not bioavailable because they are first, synthetic, and second, they need the removed fat to be absorbed. It serves no purpose.

Whey protein has been added, and you should be aware that the process used to produce whey protein creates MSG, which is known to produce hyperactivity in children and has cardiologic, neurological, circulatory, muscular, and gastrointestinal affects. The cheese cultures and enzymes used to make cheese most assuredly come from the same CAFOs as the milk. The salt used here would be table salt which has been bleached and stripped of all of the trace minerals our bodies need such as magnesium and manganese that make salt more than just a load of sodium chloride laced with chemical residue. Paprika extract is created by the same process used in making "vegetable oils" utilizing hexane or methanol to extract the oil from the seeds of the pepper for coloring. And finally, the soy lecithin, well, it's genetically modified soybean oil used as an emulsifier. This ingredient is ubiquitous.

That's a mouthful for a cheese cracker. This is only the tip of the iceberg and only one product. These ingredients and other additives just like them are lurking in all processed, refined, packaged foods. It would have been so much simpler for me to say to you, please just eat real food; but would you?

Need more evidence?

Let's talk about sugar and refined sweeteners.

Sugar is More Addictive Than Cocaine

Yes, really. It is true. This was the headline in the news recently. However, it is a little more involved than it might appear at first blush. More insidious than you know. And it's not only the sugar.

To begin, sugar cane and sugar beets are genetically modified organisms and the final product has been highly processed and all of the fiber and other nutrients removed. It is straight sucrose, which as you will see, has deleterious effects on the body.

A 2007 study[2] by French scientists at the University Bordeaux, entitled "Intense Sweetness Surpasses Cocaine Reward" concluded that, "The supranormal stimulation of [sweet] receptors by sugar-rich diets, such as those now widely available in modern societies, would generate a supranormal reward signal in the brain, with the potential to override self-control mechanisms and thus lead to addiction." A more recent study conducted by researchers at Colorado State University in 2014[3] and published in 2015, found that, "...highly processed foods, which may share characteristics with drugs of abuse (e.g. high dose, rapid rate of absorption) appear to be particularly associated with 'food addiction.'" In other words, our bodies are biologically wired to become addicted to sugar just as they are wired to become addicted to drugs, whether illicit or pharmaceutical.

What is interesting about the Colorado State University study is that it examined the glycemic load (GL) of the highly processed foods. The glycemic load includes the glycemic index which measures blood sugar spikes, but it also measures the dose of refined carbohydrates. So, for example, the sugar from a candy bar or carbohydrates from a pizza crust has been highly processed to include an increased amount of refined carbohydrates. Additionally, in highly processed foods, the water content, fiber, and protein are also stripped away; all of these cause the sugar in a natural food to be absorbed more slowly into the system, but they are not present in highly processed foods, and therefore, they are more quickly absorbed into the body, causing spikes in blood sugar, than a natural sugar from eating a piece of fruit.

Another interesting factor in the addictive quality of these foods is that rarely in natural foods do you find both sugar/carbohydrates and fat; but highly processed foods contain both and in higher doses in order to make them more palatable. These additives not only increase the "tastiness" of the food, but they also increase the potential for addictiveness and abuse.

Perhaps addiction was an unintended consequence in the early days of processed foods; if so, that is no longer the case. Food companies now engineer food to be addictive so that you will continue to eat and to buy their food. Meet Dr. Howard Moskowitz. He is a Harvard-educated psychophysicist and food industry consultant.[4] He is known as "Dr. Bliss." Early in his career he was hired by the U.S. Army to find a way to make ready-made meals more palatable. He now works for big food corporations to identify the "bliss point" of processed foods primarily through high additions of sugar, refined carbohydrates, and artificial flavorings. In other words, his job is to find the point at which the "food" is especially palatable and thus increase the likelihood of over-consumption.

In 2011, Morley Safer, of CBS's "60 Minutes" aired a segment entitled "The Flavorist: Tweaking Tastes and Creating Cravings."[5] He interviewed executives of Givaudan, a Swiss company hired by food corporations all over the world to flavor their food. Their primary job is to identify flavors, some natural, and recreate them chemically for additions to food. When Safer asked if they are trying "to create an addictive taste," one executive responded, "That's a good word." According to these executives, they engineer the flavors so that the taste doesn't linger too long on the tongue so the customer will go back for more, and more, and more. The thing that struck me most as I watched this episode was the cavalier and callous attitude of these executives and "creators of flavor." They had no remorse, no moral repulsion, seemingly no conscience; quite the opposite. They were thrilled, almost giddy, to be on the "cutting edge" of flavor engineering and their primary concern was ensuring that the flavors be enticing enough so customers would come back for more and more and more. It's all about making a buck. It was appalling!

Researchers have known for years... YEARS... that food additives and artificial flavors and colors have produced behavioral problems, especially in children. In 1964, that's 53 years ago...*fifty... three...*, Dr. Benjamin F. Feingold, a Chief Emeritus in the Allergy Department at Kaiser Permanente Hospital in San Francisco discovered the connection. When the offending foods were removed from the diet, symptoms usually abated. There are a plethora of studies on the effects of food additives and behavioral and other health issues; yet, Big Food companies continue to use them.[6]

Does this make you angry? It makes me angry. These corporations hire first rate advertising executives to craft ads meant to suggest that you can trust them with the health of your family, when in reality they do not care about your family, only their bottom line. It is up to you to be the first line of defense for your health and the health of your children. It is up to you to become armed with the truth about our food supply and the dangers lurking behind the smiling faces and happy people in the warm and fuzzy ads. The addictive nature of highly processed "food" is no accident. It is intentional. How have we become so gullible?

It's not just the chemicals in our food. Since World War II, there have been more than 85,500 chemicals introduced into the environment, from the additives in food, to skin care, to household cleaners, to air pollution, and everything in between. Every day your body is being bombarded with toxins. Some you can control; others you cannot.

You can control what you eat. You can control what types of ingredients you put on your skin, which is also an organ. When anything is absorbed through the skin, it bypasses the gut where it can be filtered, and goes straight into the blood stream. Perhaps you don't realize just how many toxins you are absorbing through your skin every day. It is seen as a barrier, and it is, but it also provides a mode of quick absorption into the bloodstream. Chemicals contained in skincare products, household cleaners, latex gloves, chemicals on clothing from manufacturing to laundry detergent to fabric softeners, anything that touches you, it can get absorbed into the body through the skin.

Your Gut has Sprung a Leak!

Do you know that 70-80% of your immune system resides in your gut? Do you also know that you have ten times more micro-organisms in your body than human cells? The bulk of those micro-organisms are in your gut and are known as the microbiome. The microbiome consists of viruses, yeast, and bacteria, which in a healthy gut have a symbiotic relationship of the good guys (mutual), the bad guys (pathogens), and the neutral guys (commensal), with the good guys and the neutral guys making up about 85% of the microbiota ensuring everything stays in top working order. It is when these guys get out of balance and the bad guys begin to outnumber the good guys that you begin to have problems and that's when you begin to feel like the witches' brew from *Macbeth*, "Double, double, toil and trouble; fire burn and cauldron bubble." If you have chronic digestive issues, you know exactly what I mean. It is when these issues are ongoing that should give us pause. It is a red flag that something is seriously wrong and it needs to be addressed.

A disruption in the microbiome, or gut flora, is at the root of all disease. Hippocrates, the Father of Medicine, thousands of years ago made that very pronouncement: All disease begins in the gut. When the gut flora become unbalanced and the pathogens outnumber the good bacteria, it causes damage to the lining of the gut wall which allows undigested food particles to escape into the blood stream which produces an immune response, which causes inflammation in the body. That is how the body protects itself from foreign invaders. Inflammation, in and of itself, is not necessarily a bad thing. If you sprain your ankle, it swells; this is the body rushing to the scene to aid in healing. God designed our bodies beautifully and with the incredible ability to heal itself. It is when the body remains in a constant state of internal inflammation and it gets stuck in fight mode that problems begin.

Inflammation begins when the intestinal wall is impaired. This condition is referred to scientifically as intestinal permeability, but it is more commonly known as "leaky gut." When the gut lining is damaged and you are constantly eating highly processed foods, ingesting chemicals, additives, over-using antibiotics, NSAIDS, proton pump inhibitors, and other medications, breathing in toxic air, applying toxic chemicals to your skin, using toxic chemical household cleaners, your body can only handle so much. It becomes overburdened. When the body remains in a constant state of inflammation, that is the beginning of degenerative diseases, autoimmune diseases, and other health conditions, all of which are on the rise. Leaky gut has been linked to:

- Alzheimer's disease
- Anxiety and depression
- Autism
- Celiac and non-celiac disease
- Hashimoto's and Grave's thyroiditis
- Rheumatoid Arthritis
- Fibromyalgia
- Crohn's disease
- Irritable Bowel Disease
- Lupus

- Metabolic Syndrome
- Multiple Sclerosis
- Parkinson's disease
- Types 1 & 2 Diabetes
- Psoriasis and other skin conditions
- Non-alcoholic fatty liver disease[7]

These are only a very few of the conditions linked to leaky gut and a disruption of the microbiome. This list is long and growing. There is much research being conducted in this field now and it is quite compelling. The conditions are not solely physical in nature, but those attributed to mental and behavioral also. There is a direct correlation between the gut and the brain. In fact, the gut is known as the second brain and the health of your gut flora is directly related to your overall health.

According to Dr. Natasha Campbell-McBride, there is no incurable disease.[8] She has written a book *Gut and Psychology Syndrome*, which deals primarily with healing the gut as it relates to children with autism and other behavioral issues; however, gut health and healing the gut is for everyone who is suffering with any type of degenerative disease or autoimmune disease, all of which are related to inflammation in the body. There is hope. Healing the gut is the key to getting well and the key to preventing disease. So why is this not more mainstream? Why doesn't your medical doctor address this? Partly because allopathic medicine compartmentalizes the body into separate systems, when in actuality, the body's systems are all related and interconnected.

Complacent and Complicit

Remember my opening question from Chapter 1: How have we become a people, a society that is so apathetic, so complacent? May I also suggest, complicit?

Researchers at UCLA have found a link between the consumption of junk food, obesity, fatigue, and complacency.[9] Yes, the researchers found that mice who ate the highly processed foods became more and more complacent over time and changing their diet for nine days to a normal diet did not measurably change their behavior, suggesting that there is no quick fix. According to the researchers, the implications for humans are that, "diet-induced obesity is a cause, rather than an effect, of laziness." In other words, a diet of highly processed food is the cause of much fatigue which leads to apathy and complacency and a whole host of health issues such as those outlined earlier.

Society has become too sick and tired to notice they are sick and tired and they have no gumption, as my grandmother would say, to do anything different. It requires too much effort to discover the problem or implement the solution. Behavioral issues abound today. Chronic diseases are on the rise.

To be sure, this is a highly complex subject, but it is important to understand that the disruption of the delicate balance of the microbiome caused by consumption of highly processed and refined foods, other forms of toxic foods, environmental toxins, the over-use of medications, leads to inflammation in the body, and if, over time, it is not addressed, leads to chronic degenerative diseases.

Dr. Price had it right 80 years ago, a "modernized western" diet full of processed foods is the cause of degenerative diseases. Big Food companies are getting rich from our complacency. However, the tide *is* turning. A revolution *is* happening. And you can be a participant and take back your health and the health of your family.

If only that were all. There are still "miles to go before [you] sleep." Let's continue down this rabbit hole and discover other ways in which our food is adulterated.

3 | They Did *What* to My Food?!

Control oil and you control nations;
control food and you control the people.
Henry Kissinger

If you want to control the food, control the seed.
Dr. Vandana Shiva

Deep within its recesses lies all of the makings of life. A quiet promise. It has the ability to grow and to nourish and to impart the life that it carries to those whom partake of its goodness. It is life. It knows nothing else, only what has been encoded into its DNA since the beginning of time. It is a gift from the Creator to you. It is a miracle waiting to be born. It is the foundation of all life. It is a seed.

And it is in danger.

Many varieties of seeds are now extinct and we don't truly know what we have lost. Hundreds of thousands of varieties are gone and we can't get them back. According to Rural Advancement Foundation International, 94% of crop varieties grown 100 years ago are now extinct.[1] This is a partial list:

> In 1903, there were 288 varieties of beets;
> today, there are 17.

In 1903, there were 497 varieties of lettuce;
today, there are 36.

In 1903, there were 307 varieties of sweet corn;
today, there are 12.

In 1903, there were 544 varieties of cabbage;
today, there are 28.

In 1903, there were 338 varieties of melon;
today, there are 27.

In 1903, there were 408 varieties of peas;
today, there are 25.

In 1903, there were 463 varieties of radish;
today, there are 27.

In 1903, there were 341 varieties of squash;
today, there are 40.

In 1903, there were 408 varieties of tomato;
today, there are 79.

In 1903, there were 285 varieties of cucumber;
today, there are 16.

Imagine it with me – 338 varieties of melon! 408 varieties of tomato! Oh, the bounty! Oh, the beauty! The myriad of colors. The plethora of shapes and sizes. The array of tastes and textures. The variety is stunning! Think of the infinite creativity of the Creator! Each seed and each plant uniquely suited to a particular location and a particular climate. Each seed containing all the nutrients your body needs to sustain life and live without disease and illness. Imagine it if you can... because imagine is all you can do... for they are gone... lost... forever. We can't get them back. Seeds are as endangered as the golden eagle or the panda or the polar bear. And the ones that are left are being adulterated.

There are laws of nature that must be obeyed. Man is not greater than God. We are created in His likeness, yes, but He alone is the perfect Creator. We cannot improve His original design.

There are companies dedicated to preserving heirloom seeds; but big agricultural corporations, the ones who grow most of the "food" in our country are not using heirloom seeds; they are using seeds which have been genetically modified and require massive amounts of chemicals to produce.

As I was traveling on vacation recently, I passed through farm land. At first blush, you might think, 'oh how pretty.' And on the one hand, it is. There is something beautiful about nature and the life it reveals; the glory of God it reveals.

However, in our culture the traditional use of land and the beauty that is the seed has been lost. Big agricultural corporations have taken over traditional farming and turned it into a monoculture enterprise.

As I passed through farm country and acre after acre after acre of the same crop, I no longer saw the beauty. Rather I saw the disaster that is modern farming which requires gallons and gallons of pesticides, herbicides, and synthetic fertilizers. The mammoth spreaders of those poisons stretch for acres and acres in continuous motion.

You see, this chemical-laden monoculture farming is destroying the land and denaturing the land; it does not contain the minerals our bodies need and it creates toxic runoff that is poisoning our rivers and streams. And that's just the beginning. The fallout is pervasive and significant. Every year, the United States uses 1 million pounds of pesticide, 750 million pounds of which are used in agriculture, the remainder being used by golf courses and home and business owners.

Brief History of Seeds

It is miserable for a farmer to be obliged to buy his Seeds; to exchange Seeds may, in some cases, be useful; but to buy them after the first year is disreputable.
– George Washington

For millennia, since the beginning of time actually, farmers and individuals have saved their seeds from year to year. As members of communities, they often swapped seeds with their neighbors. Never did they purchase seeds. In fact, seeds were considered sacred because they contained life and because they were the difference between feast and famine. Seeds were protected and cared for with diligent forethought. Those who have gone before us considered it their responsibility, obligation, and duty to humanity to save and protect seed, for they truly are a treasure worthy of protecting. In times of war and civil unrest, the first target was always the seed supply of the peoples being attacked. When the U.S. bombed Iraq during Desert Storm, it bombed the structure containing seeds that had been saved for thousands of years. Gone, forever, in one fell swoop.

As a result of this protecting of seeds for millennia, a vast diversity of seeds have been developed and adapted to the specific region and climate. In other words, the seeds which have been saved around the world over time have resulted in a variety of seeds that contain the characteristics essential for a specific region including pest control, drought, plant diseases, and other environmental conditions specific to a particular region. This process, coupled with sustainable farming practices, has served humanity very well over thousands of years.

Early in America's history, Thomas Jefferson, in 1793, drafted the first patent statute which stated that living organisms were considered to be the 'common heritage' of mankind. In other words, seeds were not considered to be patentable. It is common practice and belief around the world that nature cannot be patented.

In an effort to strengthen economic development, the United States Department of Agriculture was created in 1862. As will soon become apparent, nothing good ever comes from the government getting involved. The initial efforts by the USDA centered around a program of seed distribution. The government gathered seeds from around the world and distributed them to farmers across the country.

In the early 20th century, the USDA, land-grant universities, state experiment stations, and other publicly funded institutions began to conduct more systematic testing and breeding of new crop varieties. This practice ushered in the process of hybridization (explained more fully in the next section) and what was referred to as "high-yielding" varieties of crops.

With the rise of industrialism, the wealthy industrialist thought it was a good idea to turn farming and hybridization of seeds into a commodity to be bought and sold on the stock market and measured in spread sheets. This ushered in the role of the private sector into the story of seeds. Why were hybridized seeds so enticing for industrialist? Because hybrid seeds do not reproduce true to type from year to year, and they therefore must be purchased anew yearly.

Enter the Plant Patent Act of 1930 (PPA) which allowed for the patenting of *asexually* propagated plants, meaning plants reproduced via budding, cutting, and grafting. Most importantly was what Congress excluded from the PPA: *sexually* reproduced plants which include almost all food-producing plants. This exclusion reflected the belief of farmers for millennia and the belief of George Washington and Thomas Jefferson: neither private nor public entities should be entrusted with a monopoly control over our food supply – the seed.[2]

Alas, man continues to do what is right in his own mind. In 1970, Congress passed the Plant Variety Protection Act (PVPA). This Act allowed the USDA to confer Certificates of Protection for "novel" *sexually* producing plant varieties. The marketer had exclusive rights to a "protected" variety for 18 years (later amended to 20 years). However, there were two exemptions provided in the Certifications: one, the farmers must be allowed to save seeds for replanting; and two, patented varieties must be made available for researchers. In spite of these exemptions, this Act was to become Pandora's Box, opening the way for genetically engineered seeds owned by chemical companies and pharmaceutical companies, and the stripping of the rights of farmers and researchers to save seed and to perform research on the different varieties.[3]

In 1980, in a landmark 5-4 decision by the Supreme Court in *Diamond v. Chakrabarty*, the court held for the first time that living organisms, specifically in this case genetically modified bacterium, could be patented. The Supreme Court ruled that because those petitioning for the patent had introduced new genetic material within the bacterium cell, in effect, it had produced something that was not part of nature. This and subsequent judicial decisions paved the way for the patenting of *sexually* reproducing plants and control of those seeds by private chemical companies.[4]

Why does this matter? It matters because farmers are no longer in control of the seed (food) supply, rather the chemical companies that own the seeds control the seed (food) supply. Farmers are forced to purchase new seeds each year at higher and higher costs, along with more and more chemical fertilizers, pesticides, and herbicides that are required to be sprayed on these seeds. And if that were not enough, they face an avalanche of lawsuits for inadvertently "saving" seeds or because GE seeds were found in the fields of organic farmers due to natural pollination. Often, these lawsuits put these independent farmers out of business and in enormous legal debt for something that was beyond their control. Independent research is prohibited. Food freedom was slowly stripped away from the people.

The result: the multi-million dollar chemical companies, Monsanto, Bayer (these two are in the process of merging), Syngenta (recently bought out by ChemChina), Dow, BASF, and DuPont, own and control 94% of the world's seeds.

Defining Genetically Engineered (GE) and Genetically Modified (GM) Foods.

Before I dive into an explanation of genetically engineered foods, let me explain the difference between genetically engineered and genetically modified organisms.

It is commonplace to use the terms GE and GMO interchangeably; in fact, the USDA uses the term GMO to describe both; however, they are two distinct processes. Genetically modified organisms have been around for millennia and it is more commonly referred to as hybridization. It is the process by which cross-pollination occurs thereby creating a new "breed" of plant to acquire a particular trait; it is done within a species: one type of tomato is bred with another type of tomato. This can be done intentionally or by naturally occurring processes inherent in nature, in which case those seeds are referred to as open-pollinated, and they can reproduce exact replicas from year to year from saved seeds; this initial process takes several years to complete.

Hybridized seeds that are genetically modified within one generation are not open-pollinated, and therefore cannot reproduce the next year. For instance, a seed company hybridizes a particular variety of squash. When you purchase a packet of those seeds from your local garden store, the seeds produced by the squash you grow that year cannot be saved to produce the same plant the following year. If those seeds by chance produce a crop, they will not have the same characteristics and they will be less productive and less viable; in other words, they will not grow true to type. This is advantageous for seed companies in that the farmer must purchase new seeds each year. This is a large expense.

Gardeners have been "breeding" plants for thousands of years and the process takes several years to achieve the desired result. This is typically performed to create certain traits such as drought tolerant or disease tolerant plants specific to the region in which the gardener lives and grows his plants. This is usually done within a species: one type of tomato is bred with another type of tomato to attain a certain characteristic. Again, the desired result takes years to achieve and once achieved, those seeds can be saved from year to year to produce those plants with the same results. Hybridized plants, on the other hand, cannot be saved and must be recreated in the "lab" each year and sold to farmers and home-gardeners yearly. In 19th Century horticulture, hybrids were referred to as "yoles" or vegetable mules, because they were unable to reproduce.

Hybridization ushered in the modern era and what is referred to as high intensity industrialized monoculture. This high intensity monoculture then ushered in the need for large quantities of nitrogen fertilizer[5] (we had to do something with those stockpiles of nitrogen left over from WWII), which led to the development of a system designed to use high amounts of petro-chemical fertilizers. In brief, modern farming practices were developed to line the pockets of the petroleum and chemical industries, not as a means of feeding the world.

Bottom line, current hybridized (GM) and genetically engineered (GE) seeds are developed to create extensive use of chemicals, fertilizers, herbicides, and fungicides.

Let's look at corn as an example. Corn is both GM and GE (it is also a grain, not a vegetable). Nitrogen is added to the soil so that crop rotation is no longer needed; but the corn plant must be able to withstand the overload of nitrogen in the soil, so it is genetically modified with that trait. However, the weeds love the nitrogen, and in order to control the weeds, copious amounts of herbicide must be sprayed to keep them in check. In order to do that, the corn must also be genetically engineered to withstand the herbicide sprayed on the weeds and it must also be able to stand in spite of the high levels of nitrogen in the soil. The absence of crop rotation, the presence of herbicides and excess nitrogen create a perfect storm. It is a breeding ground for insects, which requires pesticides, which requires that the corn be genetically engineered to resist pests.

It is a vicious cycle.

It bears repeating that the use of GM and GE seeds has created a huge market for all of the "-cides" and fertilizers. Over 5 billion tons (or 10 trillion pounds) of pesticides are used worldwide every year. Conventional farmers spray 10-15 different chemical products on their crops three times a year. The use of Roundup® has increased 1000-fold in the last 20 years since the inception of GE crops in the 1990s. As with the rise of anti-bacterial resistance, so is there a rise in the need for chemicals that are stronger than the current glyphosate in Roundup. Because weeds are becoming resistant to the active ingredient in Roundup, glyphosate, Monsanto, the maker of Roundup, is making a new, stronger product called 2-4-D which was an element in Agent Orange, also created by Monsanto. The drifts from this product can wipe out *all* plant life. We have taken a path that has far-reaching and irrevocable consequences.[6]

Genetically modified organisms can be anything, not just plants. Scientists have taken the silk protein gene from a spider and inserted into the DNA of a goat so that when the goat is milked, it produces a silk protein from which bullet-proof vests can be made. Scientists have inserted the gene which produces the hide of a cow and inserted into the DNA of a pig to give the pigs cowhide. They have also taken human genes and inserted them into corn to create spermicide. Once this genetic code is created, it cannot be reversed. Is this really the path we want to go down?

Genetic Engineering of Plants[7]

Please be aware that although I use the term "genetic engineering" throughout this discussion because it is the appropriate and most descriptive term, I am referring to what the USDA, most companies, organizations, and consumers refer to as genetically modified organisms (GMOs).

In simple terms, the process of genetic engineering of plants is the process of taking the gene (DNA) of one species, such as bacteria, virus, or pesticide, and inserting it into the gene (DNA) of another species, a plant such as corn. Sounds appetizing, doesn't it? There are two primary types of genetic engineering. The first is herbicide-tolerate (HT) and the second is built-in pesticide.

This is not an extension of natural breeding of plants. In genetic engineering, a single gene from a particular species is removed and inserted into the DNA of another species. In essence, this is akin to a cow mating with a squash; this cannot and does not happen naturally. This process transfers genes across natural boundaries that have been in existence for millennia. As parents, we set boundaries for our children for their protection. The same holds true for all species. These boundaries are in place for a reason.

Herbicide Tolerant

Herbicide tolerant crops are just as their name implies. Plants engineered with this trait can withstand being sprayed with herbicide, specifically Monsanto's Roundup, 2-4-D, or Bayer's Liberty Herbicide. (When farmers buy Monsanto or Bayer's Liberty Link seeds, they must also buy the herbicides created by those companies for use on those seeds.)

How is it that herbicides can be sprayed on plants and they do not die? Scientists at Monsanto discovered bacteria growing in a chemical waste dump near their Roundup factory. When they realized this bacterium could resist the main ingredient in Roundup, glyphosate, the scientists set out to identify the gene responsible for the resistance. Once they isolated that gene, they removed it from the bacteria and inserted it into the DNA of plant cells.

They do not do this one cell at a time, rather they place thousands of cells in a petri dish, load a "gun" and shoot the bacteria gene into the dish. In order to determine which "transgenes" implanted into the DNA of the cells in the petri dish, the scientists insert an antibiotic resistant marker prior to the gene insertion. The cells are then covered with antibiotics, which kills all of the cells except those in which the transgene has implanted into the DNA, making those cells antibiotic resistant. The remaining cells are then cloned into a plant which is both herbicide tolerant as well as antibiotic resistant.

Glyphosate, the active ingredient in Roundup, was originally patented as a broad spectrum chelator. Chelation is the process of binding ions and molecules to metal ions. In other words, the metal ions are trapped or encapsulated in the chelation process. In 1974, glyphosate was patented as an herbicide.

Roundup kills weeds by making the nutrients unavailable to the plant, which weakens the plant, which in turn promotes disease in the soil, ultimately killing the plant. Plants that are herbicide tolerant can be sprayed with Roundup without dying; however, these plants are nutrient-deficient. The animals that eat these plants are, therefore, nutrient deficient, as are the humans who eat the animals who eat the nutrient-depleted plants. Also, the plants humans are eating are also nutrient-depleted plants, and thus our bodies are deficient as well.

If that were not enough, the residue of glyphosate that ends up in our bodies chelates the nutrients we do consume. What this means is that the nutrients chelated by the glyphosate in our bodies are trapped and moved out of the body during elimination, leaving us nutrient deficient, further contributing to the development of disease.

As stated earlier, to make matters worse, these herbicide tolerant crops are no longer responding to Roundup, so Monsanto is using the same method to engineer crops to be resistant to 2-4-D, an element contained in Agent Orange.

Pesticide-Producing

Pesticide-producing crops, again, are as their name implies; every cell of the plant produces its own pesticide, so that when an insect bites the plant it ingests a pesticide which causes the stomach of the insect to break open, killing the insect.

To create a plant that produces its own pesticide, scientists take a gene from a naturally occurring bacteria in the soil that produces its own pesticide, specifically, *Bacillus thuringiensis* (*Bt*). This toxin is used in organic farming as a spray; it washes off and is biodegradable. Once this *Bt* toxin is inserted in a plant, it is encapsulated and concentrated thousands of times greater than the spray form and it is intentionally designed to be more toxic.

The process for creating this plant is the same as the process for creating the herbicide tolerant plant. Corn, cotton, and soy are the types of plants that are genetically engineered to produce the *Bt* toxin. In fact, corn is a registered pesticide and 93% of the corn produced in the United States is *Bt* corn.

Following is a list of crops which have been registered by the International Service for the Acquisition of Agri-Biotech Applications. The term "varieties" means specific registrations; so for Alfalfa, for instance, there are five different types of alfalfa plants that have been genetically engineered and registered.

CROP	GM/GE TRAIT(S)	USE
Alfalfa (*Medicago sativa*) (5 varieties)	Herbicide Tolerant Antibiotic Resistance Altered Lignin Production	Animal Feed
Apple (*malus Domestica*) (3 varieties) "Arctic Golden Delicious" "Arctic" "Arctic Fuji Apple"	Antibiotic Resistance Non-browning phenotype	Food
Argentina Canola (*Brassica napus*) (39 varieties)	Herbicide Tolerant Antibiotic Resistance Modified oil/ fatty acid Phytase Production	Cooking Oil Animal Feed
Chicory (*Cichorium intybus*) (3 varieties)	Herbicide Tolerant Antibiotic Resistance Male Sterility	Not commercially available in the U.S. as of this writing

Cotton (*Gossypium hirsutum L.*) (58 varieites)	Herbicide Tolerant Antibiotic Resistance *Bt* toxin producing 2-4-D Tolerant	Animal Feed Cottonseed Oil – used to make vegetable oils
Eggplant (*Solanum melongena*) (1 variety)	*Bt* Producing Antibiotic Resistance	Not commercially available in the U.S. as of this writing
Flax, linseed (*Linum usitatissumum L.*)	Herbicide Tolerant Antibiotic Resistance Nopaline Synthesis	Not commercially available in the U.S. as of this writing
Maize (Corn) (*Zea mays L.*) (196 varieties) Most varieties contain more than one modification	*Bt* Producing Herbicide Tolerant Antibiotic Resistance Modified Amylase Mannose metabolism Drought stress tolerance Male sterility 2-4-D Tolerance	Livestock and poultry feed High fructose corn syrup Other sweeteners food Corn oil Starch Cereal and other food ingredients Alcohol Fuel / ethanol Other industrial uses
Melon (*Cucumis melo*) Cantelope (2 varities)	Antibiotic Resistance Delayed ripening	Not commercially available in the U.S. as of this writing
Papaya (*Carica papaya*) (4 varieties)	Viral disease resistance Antibiotic resistance Visual marker	Food

Plum (*Prunus domestica*) (1 variety)	Viral disease resistance Antibiotic resistance Visual marker	Not commercially available in the U.S. as of this writing
Polish Canola (*Brassica rapa*) (1 variety)	Herbicide Tolerant	Not commercially available in the U.S. as of this writing
Potato (*Solanum tuiberosum L.*) (47 varieties)	*Bt* Producing Antibiotic Resistance Modified Starch Non-Bruising	Food
Rice (*Oryza sativa L.*) (7 varieties)	*Bt* Producing Antibiotic Resistance Herbicide Tolerant	Not commercially available in the U.S. as of this writing
Soybean (*Glycine max L.*) (36 varieties)	Herbicide Tolerant *Bt* Toxin Producing Antibiotic Resistance Modified fatty acid Visual Marker	Livestock and animal feed Aquatic culture Vegetable oil High oleic acid Soymilk, soy sauce, tofu and other food uses Lecithin Pet food Biodiesel fuel Adhesives and building materials Printer ink Other industrial uses

Squash (*Cucurbita pepo*) (2 varieties) Crookneck Zucchini	Antibiotic Resistance Viral Disease Resistance	Food
Sugar Beet (*Beta vulgaris*) (3 varieties)	Herbicide Tolerant Antibiotic Resistance Visual marker	Food Animal feed
Sugar Cane (*Saccharum sp.*) (3 varieties)	Antibiotic Resistance Drought stress tolerance	Food
Sweet Pepper (*Capsicum annuum*) (1 variety)	Viral disease resistance	Not commercially available in the U.S. as of this writing
Tomato (*Lycopersicon esculentum*) (11 varieties)	*Bt* Toxin producing Antibiotic Resistance Delayed Ripening Delayed Fruit Softening	Not commercially available in the U.S. as of this writing
Wheat (*Triticum aestivum*) United States – reportedly stopped pursuing regulatory process. It has been reported that GE wheat has been found growing in the Pacific Northwest near where the trials were conducted.	Herbicide Tolerant	HOWEVER: Chemically modified wheat which is herbicide tolerant is used exclusively.

Also, genetically modified salmon have been developed and are available commercially in the United States. The salmon have been genetically engineered to grow twice as fast as conventional salmon. Environmentalists claim the transgenic salmon could escape from fish farm pens and interbreed with wild salmon, threatening the species. There are many other fruits, vegetables, grasses, and animals which are undergoing genetic engineering testing. Genetically engineered Kentucky Bluegrass, designed to withstand massive amounts of Roundup, has escaped trial fields and contaminated neighboring lands. This could eventually threaten the organic and pastured-beef industry.[8] This must end!

Wheat, while not modified by "genetic engineering" is modified through the use of chemicals. The process is called chemical mutagenesis (CM) and can be achieved with chemicals, gama rays, or sodium azide, a toxic compound and hazardous material. As with genetic engineering, chemical mutagenesis cannot control where mutations in the DNA will occur. Sodium azide is a toxic industrial compound and if ingested, that person should not receive CPR because the person administering the CRP could die. If the person who ingested the sodium azide vomits, the waste should not be washed down the drain because it could explode. And this is what they use to modify wheat? Is it any wonder that the rate of Celiac disease has doubled in the last 20 years, not to mention the ubiquitous incidence of intestinal permeability?

Man has done what is right in his own mind.

Three questions beg for answers; there are certainly more than three questions that require answers, but there are three significant burning questions that need to be explored:

- How did our government allow this?
- How do these organisms impact our health?
- Can it be fixed?

The Revolving Door

Scientists at the Food and Drug Administration (FDA) had serious concerns about the use of antibiotic resistant genes; these were the best of the best scientists in the country. "IT WOULD BE A SERIOUS HEALTH HAZARD TO INTRODUCE A GENE THAT CODES FOR ANTIBIOTIC RESISTANCE INTO THE NORMAL FLORA OF THE GENERAL POPULATION." (Emphasis is from the original document, i.e., it was originally written in all caps).[9] Additionally, they were concerned that the process of genetic engineering could result in unintended consequences. In fact, in the medical officer's summary these scientists stated that they strongly recommended that long-term studies be conducted prior to the introduction of these plants into the population for consumption, issuing warnings that these foods could have serious side effects such as allergens, toxins, new diseases, and nutritional problems.

The Center for Veterinary Medicine (CVM) warned that the meat and dairy products sold from animals fed a diet of genetically modified feed could be toxic. Gerald Guest, Direct of the CVM, stated, "Animal feeds derived from genetically modified plants present unique animal and food safety concerns.... I would urge you to eliminate statements that suggest that the lack of information can be used as evidence for no regulatory concern." Additionally, numerous other departments and organizations issued the same or similar warnings.

FDA microbiologist, Louis Pribyl, argued that, "This is the [biotech] industry's pet idea, namely that there are no unintended effects that will raise the FDA's level of concern. But time and time again, there is no data to back up their contention." He went on the say, "What has happened to the scientific elements of this [policy statement] document? Without a sound scientific base to rest on, this becomes a broad, general, 'What do I have to do to avoid trouble'-type document.... It will look like and probably be just a political document.... It reads very pro-industry, especially in the area of unintended effects." Despite these warnings, on May 29, 1992, the FDA issued a policy statement which read:

> "The agency is not aware of any information showing that foods derived by these new methods differ from other foods in any meaningful or uniform way."

This policy statement is still in effect today. In essence, this stance by the FDA allowed Monsanto and other biotech companies to flood the market with genetically engineered foods without any testing. The agency charged with protecting citizens from harmful substances has given the biotech industry *carte blanc* to do as it pleases.

How did this happen? How is it that the warnings from the best and brightest scientists in the country are ignored by the agency created to protect us?

This happened because the man in charge of FDA policy at the time was Monsanto's former attorney and later their vice-president, Michael Taylor. He was the first of many biotech industry executives to hold public office in federal departments in charge of food and agriculture.

BIOTECH INDUSTRY		GOVERNMENT
Former Monsanto Attorney and then Vice-President of Monsanto	Michael Taylor	FDA Deputy Commissioner for Food 1991 Food Safety Czar 2010
Awarded "Governor of Year 2001" by Biotech Industry Association; his law firm defended Monsanto in a Supreme Court case	Tom Vilsack	U.S. Secretary of Agriculture 2009

BIOTECH INDUSTRY		GOVERNMENT
Director, Danforth Center (Monsanto)	Roger Beachy	Director, USDA, NIFA 2009
Board of Director Monsanto subsidiary	Ann Venemann	U.S. Secretary of Agriculture 2001
Monsanto Scientist of Bovine Growth Hormone (rBGH)	Margaret Miller	FDA Branch Chief that evaluated rBGH 1989
Vice-President Government and Public Affairs, Monsanto	Linda Fisher	EPA Deputy Administrator 2001

The George H.W. Bush White House instructed the FDA to promote the biotech industry and thus created the position for Michael Taylor, which enabled Monsanto and other biotech companies to release into the market any GM crops they pleased without any oversight by the FDA. Years later, the Obama administration rehired Michael Taylor as the FDA US Food Safety Czar. This is akin to the fox guarding the hen house.

The biotech industry has very deep pockets and many lobbyists to do their bidding, effectively squashing a bill to require labeling of GMOs. Additionally, Monsanto and the other biotech companies pushing GE plants have paid for the "science." They have funneled millions of dollars into universities (Cornell, Harvard, University of Illinois, University of Georgia, Danforth Center, University of California/Riverside, Tuskegee University, Pennsylvania State), and paid the scientists and administrative officials to produce the results that they needed and to push GMOs,[10] all the while dismissing the science that demonstrated that at the very least these organisms required further testing. Not one human trial has been performed in this county. There are laws in place that require testing of new technologies, such as GE crops, before entering the marketplace; however, the FDA decided that these crops were considered generally accepted as safe based on the self-imposed tests of the biotech industry itself, while ignoring the warnings of scientists from all over the world.[11]

If genetically modified organisms are safe, as the FDA, EPA, USDA, and the biotech industry claim, then why not label them? Why spend millions of dollars to defeat a bill before Congress requiring GMO labeling? What do they have to hide?

Apparently, a lot.

In 2015, the International Agency for Research on Cancer (IARC), a department within the World Health Organization (WHO) determined that glyphosate is a "probable human carcinogen" and likely to cause non-Hodgkin's lymphoma and other hematopoietic cancers (cancers such as leukemia and myeloma).

In 2016, hundreds of individuals filed lawsuits against Monsanto alleging that they or their loved ones have non-Hodgkin's lymphoma caused by Roundup and its active ingredient, glyphosate. As a result of the release of certain documents, it has been revealed that Monsanto has been pushing a lot of fake science on the public. Documents obtained pursuant to these lawsuits "suggest that Monsanto had ghostwritten research that was later attributed to academics and indicated that a senior official at the Environmental Protection Agency (EPA) had worked to quash a review of Roundup's main ingredient, glyphosate, which was to have been conducted by the United States Health and Human Services." In other documents released pursuant to the court order, this same senior EPA official, Jess Rowland, told Monsanto that, "If I can kill this, I should get a medal" referring to blocking the review by the United States Health and Human Services.[12]

In fact, Monsanto does not allow their seeds to undergo third party testing. Remember that one of the exceptions under the Plant Variety Protection Act of 1970 required that seeds be made available for third-party testing. Pursuant to a plethora of lawsuits filed by Monsanto over the years, now only universities that receive special grants from Monsanto and Monsanto-appointed scientists may test their seeds. Other scientists who have obtained seeds and tested them and whose findings are diametrically opposed to those of Monsanto, have had their careers ruined, lost their jobs, and had their reputation discredited. In short, their lives have been destroyed.[13]

In another document released pursuant to these lawsuits, a long time, 30 year toxicologist for the EPA, Marion Copley, wrote a letter to Jess Rowland in 2013. This scientist, who was dying with cancer at the time, urged him to come clean and to stop playing "your political conniving games with the science to favor the registrants [i.e., the chemical companies, including Monsanto]. For once do the right thing and don't make decisions based on how it affects your bonus." She goes on to accuse Rowland and another EPA official, Anna Lowit, of intimidation of staff members of the Cancer Assessment Review Committee (CARC) and of changing Hazard Identification Assessment Review Committee (HIARC) and Hazard and Science Policy Committee (HASPOC) final reports to reflect favorably on the chemical industry.[14]

Additionally, in this letter Copley outlines 14 different processes on how glyphosate, originally designed as a chelator, are involved in tumor formation and points out that any of these processes individually can cause tumor formation, but that "glyphosate causes all of them simultaneously:"

1. Chelators inhibit apoptosis, the process by which our bodies kill tumor cells

2. Chelators are endocrine disruptors, involved in tumorigenesis

3. Glyphosate induces lymphocyte proliferation

4. Glyphosate induces free radical formation

5. Chelators inhibit free radical scavenging enzymes requiring Zn, Mn or Cu for activity (i.e. SODs)

6. Chelators bind zinc, necessary for immune system function

7. Glyphosate is genotoxic, a key cancer mechanism

8. Chelators inhibit DNA repair enzymes requiring metal cofactors

9. Chelators bind Ca, Zn, Mg, etc. to make foods deficient for these essential nutrients

10. Chelators bind calcium necessary for calcineurin-mediated immune response

11. Chelators often damage the kidneys or pancreas, as glyphosate does, a mechanism to tumor formation

12. Kidney/pancreas damage can lead to clinical chemistry changes to favor tumor growth

13. Glyphosate kills bacteria in the gut and the gastrointestinal system in 80% of the immune system

14. Chelators suppress the immune system making the body susceptible to tumors[15]

The United States Department of Agriculture (USDA) routinely tests food for pesticide residue, but they do not test for glyphosate. However, there had been plans to begin testing high fructose corn syrup; but suddenly, those plans changed and the USDA will not test for glyphosate contamination after conversations with officials at the EPA.[16] The collusion between Monsanto, the chemical industry at large, and various governmental agencies, especially the EPA, runs deep and wide and long. The agency created to protect citizens is in the business of protecting its officials and their bonuses and cushy positions.

I don't know about you, but this makes me angry. It makes me angry that they have gotten away with it for so long and it makes me angry that these companies are more concerned with their bottom line than with the health of humanity. Truly, it is a red flag when the largest chemical companies in the world own the majority of the seeds used to feed the people. Is it me, or is that an oxymoron to you? Why would we allow chemical companies charge over our food supply?

I will leave that question for you to ponder.

Health Consequences

Whether we and our politicians know it or not, Nature is
party to all our deals and decisions, and she has more votes, a
longer memory, and a sterner sense of justice than we do.
Wendell Berry

Aside from scientific studies not made public by the FDA, USDA, EPA, Monsanto, and other biotech companies, anecdotal evidence, and causal and correlational relationships, there are five considerations when looking at health problems associated with genetically engineered organisms.

First, as mentioned earlier, the process of creating genetically engineered crops may create unintended changes in the DNA. Insertion of the transgene can cause changes in the sequencing of the DNA, or it can delete native genes. Native genes can be turned off permanently or turned on permanently. This can cause an overproduction of protein which may result in the gene being an allergen, a toxin, a carcinogen, or an anti-nutrient, which blocks the absorption of minerals. Additionally, hundreds, if not thousands, of mutations can occur. There is much collateral damage as a result of the process of creating the genetically engineered crop (or animal).

This means that proteins that are generally harmless can become extremely hazardous proteins. GE soy contains seven times the amount of trypsin inhibitor (an allergen) than non-GE soy. The cooking process does not destroy these allergens. (Soy should be avoided for a variety of reasons, this is only one!). This same principle holds true for GE corn.

The second potential problem is that the intended protein, produced by the inserted gene, may be harmful. The *Bt* toxin inserted into corn, soybean, and cotton, has been found in the intestinal tract of mice where they suffered significant tissue damage. In addition, the mice developed an immune system response to the *Bt* which resulted in a multiple chemical sensitivity. *Bt* spray has been shown to affect humans when sprayed, even causing hospitalization. However, the *Bt* in the crop, itself, is more problematic and hazardous than the spray.

In India, farmers of *Bt* cotton developed terrible skin rashes and many had to be hospitalized. After the *Bt* cotton was harvested, thousands of sheep that were grazing on the plants died. Investigation into these deaths revealed that there were black patches in the intestine, liver, and bile ducts. The keepers of these sheep indicated that they saw instances of nasal discharge, dulled senses, diarrhea, and coughing. Other livestock also suffered skin problems as a result of the *Bt* toxin in the cotton.

If that were not enough, in 2008 because the harvest associated with the *Bt* cotton was dismal, even though Monsanto claims that GE crops can withstand drought conditions better than indigenous varities, the farmers (in India) were not able to pay back the loans they acquired to purchase the GE seeds and the chemicals required for the seeds. As a result, 125,000 farmers committed suicide by drinking the pesticides they were required to purchase from Monsanto.

There are other similar stories from farmers around the world; animal deaths, even some unexplained human deaths as a result of using *Bt* crops.

In 2013, a Canadian study of 31 pregnant women found that 93% of the women had *Bt* toxin in their blood; it was found in 80% of the fetuses of these women. Since the blood-brain barrier is not yet formed in these fetuses, it was suggested that the *Bt* toxin could have passed into the brain of these fetuses causing unknown consequences. The authors of the study suggested that the toxin was present in the meat and milk consumed by the women.

In 2012, a study reported in the *Journal of Applied Toxicology* found that the *Bt* toxin from corn also broke open holes in the intestinal wall of human cells, causing the intestines to leak. The authors suggested that this could be one cause of gastrointestinal permeability or "leaky gut" and other digestive disorders which are on the rise. (See Appendix for list of ingredients made with GE corn.)

The third cause of problems with genetically engineered crops is that the protein created by the inserted gene may be different than it was intended. The transgene sequence determines the amino acids of protein produced. Therefore, if the sequence changes in any way, so does the protein. The sequence can mutate or truncate; it can rearrange; it can be read differently; and it can produce multiple proteins. All of these sequence changes have occurred.

Laboratories in France and Belgium tested the sequence of the transgene of six different genetically engineered crops and found that the sequence was entirely different than that which was registered by the biotech company with the International Service for the Acquisition of Agri-Biotech Applications (ISAAA). There were also instances where the transgene sequence was different even between the two laboratories. This implies that along with the transgene being unstable, there are varied ways in which the sequence can rearrange.

In addition, the transgene, even if it is identical to what was intended, the proteins can fold and change shapes, which affect its function within the cell. Multiple proteins folded together can cause a myriad of harmful problems. Some of these folded proteins are responsible for mad cow disease as well as the human variant of that disease, along with Alzheimer's and Parkinson's disease. There any many other ways that a protein can fold which changes the way it is expressed causing significant problems including respiratory problems, allergies, lupus, immune system response, and inflammatory bowel disease, to name just a few.

The fourth problem that genetic engineering of crops produces is an increase in the use of herbicides and herbicide residue on the crops engineered to be resistant to the herbicide, which we then consume. Glyphosate, the active ingredient in Roundup, has properties which cause endocrine disruption, along with the probability of it being a human carcinogen and responsible for non-Hodgkin's lymphoma and other hepatic cancers.

From 1996 to 2011, herbicide use in the United States increased by 527 million pounds. While the use of insecticidal chemicals decreased with the use of *Bt* crops, the amount of pesticide produced by the crops themselves far outweighs the amount of insecticide use they have displaced. Poultry fed *Bt* corn die at twice the rate as poultry feed non-GM corn. Other livestock health has suffered also as a result of genetically engineered corn, alfalfa, and soy.

The fifth potential problem with genetically engineered crops is the possibility that the transgene inserted into the plant may transfer to our gut bacteria and into the DNA of our cells. You could be producing pesticides in your gut. Remember the Canadian study of the pregnant women mentioned above? Remember I also mentioned that normally there is a natural barrier between species that prevents different species from crossing? When we eat vegetables, the structure of the plant cell is different from the structure of our cells and the sequencing of the DNA is different which prevents the plant's DNA cells from integrating with ours. The process of genetic engineering removes that barrier.

Genetically engineered plants contain a bacteria which has been inserted. Our bodies contain bacteria; in fact, bacterial cells outnumber our human cells 10:1. With the insertion of bacteria into plant cells, the process of genetic engineering itself removes any barriers against transmission, so the possibility that those transgenes can be transferred to our cells increases. Not only that, but these transgene bacteria are living, functioning transgenes residing and possibly colonizing in our gut and potentially transforming the DNA of our cells, even long after we stop eating genetically engineered foods.

A human feeding study of seven individuals with a colostomy bag found that the Roundup Ready soy transgene did, in fact, transfer into the bacteria living inside the intestines and these transgenes continued to function, disproving the biotech industry's claim that these genes are destroyed with digestive enzymes. They not only survived the stomach, but they also survived passage through the lower intestines. Perhaps more importantly, present in the gut bacteria of three out of the seven volunteers was the transgene from soy that had integrated into the DNA *before* they had their test meal, suggesting that it was acquired and integrated into their gut bacteria from a previous meal. This study clearly demonstrates that the transgenes from genetically modified crops do transfer into gut bacteria and they do continue to function.

There are several aspects of the genetically engineered crops that can transfer into our gut microbiome. There is a "promoter" gene which is inserted; its function is to turn the inserted gene "on." This promoter gene can inadvertently turn on unintended genes and cause an over-production of protein which can be allergenic, toxic, carcinogenic, or act as an anti-nutrient inside our gut bacteria or the DNA of our cells.

Antibiotic resistant genes can transfer. The scientists at the FDA and around the globe sternly warned officials in the early 1990s that this could be a serious problem leading to widespread antibiotic resistance. Unfortunately, their prediction has come true. We are now faced with the threat that deadly microbes will outpace the science to combat them.

It has already been proven that Roundup Ready transgenes can transfer to humans as well as the *Bt* toxin gene which has been found in the blood of pregnant women and their fetuses. Could our gut bacteria turn into a pesticide-producing factory? Additionally, there are virus genes found in Hawaiian papaya, zucchini, and crookneck squash that have the potential to transfer to the human genome or they could suppress the body's own defenses, and there is a possibility that these transgenes are also toxic.

With regard to Roundup and Liberty Link, it is more than just the active ingredient, glyphosate. The inert ingredients, surfactants, play a role in toxicity also. These surfactants open the pores and drive the glyphosate into the plant. It also drives it into our bodies. These inert ingredients have been found to be more toxic than the glyphosate, and when added to the glyphosate, they are thousands of times more toxic. Because it gets driven into the plant, it cannot be washed off; 80-85% stays in the plant and it is sprayed on approximately 100 different crops before they are harvested.

These toxic chemicals are in our air, our blood, our babies' blood, our urine, our surface water, and our ground water. It has created an environmental plight and a perfect storm. The Institute for Responsible Technology has compiled a list of charts demonstrating the rise in chronic diseases with the introduction of glyphosate and genetically modified organisms. Because there have been no complex, long-term human studies, these charts serve as a correlation; however, if there is found to be a relationship it can be supported by these charts.[17]

As stated earlier, genetically engineered soy has seven times higher amount of trypsin inhibitor which is a known allergen; trypsin digests protein. When the digestion of protein is inhibited, it can lead to a cascade of disorders.

In 2009, the American Academy of Environmental Medicine performed animal feeding studies and looked at the problems that were occurring in animals that were being fed genetically engineered crops compared to those that were not fed genetically engineered crops. They found an a sundry of problems: gastrointestinal, reproductive, immune system problems, accelerated aging, organ damage, and problems with cholesterol and insulin. Any of that sound familiar?

Scientists are now claiming that glyphosate is the most chronically toxic chemical on the plant because of its ubiquitous use and how devastating it can be to our health. A study in 2013 linked glyphosate to heart disease, obesity, diabetes, cancer, reproductive disorders, gastrointestinal problems, Alzheimer's, Parkinson's, multiple sclerosis, aggression, depression, gluten sensitivity, kidney failure, non-Hodgkin's lymphoma, and endocrine disruption.

Again, glyphosate is a chelator and as such it binds with minerals making them unavailable to our bodies. Minerals operate as keys and locks which control all of the functions in our body. Mineral deficiency is a major cause of disease. Also, glyphosate is a broad-spectrum antibiotic, meaning it kills the bad as well as the good bacteria, which promotes an overgrowth of pathogens, or negative bacteria, in our intestinal tract, which in turn creates a condition known as small intestine bacterial overgrowth (SIBO). This promotes the production of caustic gas which damages the lining of the intestinal wall, negatively affects enzyme production which is needed to digest proteins, and it damages the microvilli, tiny hair-like cells lining the inside of the intestines. When these are damaged, it leads to intestinal permeability, or leaky gut.

If that were not enough, glyphosate also blocks the metabolic pathways which produce L-tryptophan which is needed for our bodies to produce serotonin and melatonin. When serotonin production is disrupted, it results in mood and behavior disorders as well as problems with insulin production by signaling to the body that it is not full; then we overeat. Yet, the body is starved of minerals, so it continues to be hungry. It destroys enzymes needed for detoxification, thereby making a toxic environment even more toxic.

And the vicious cycle continues.

Can It Be Fixed?

The ecological teaching of the Bible is simply inescapable:
God made the world because He wanted it made. He thinks
the world is good, and He loves it. It is His world; He has
never relinquished title to it. And He has never revoked the
conditions, bearing on His gift to us of the use of it, that
oblige us to take excellent care of it.
Wendell Berry

The biotech industry wants to genetically engineer the remainder of the food supply, the fish, and livestock, as well as trees. The damage caused by these organisms in the environment is irreversible. It cannot be decontaminated. Once the gene pool is genetically engineered, it cannot be reversed. That trials of other crops have escaped their trial fields and infected other lands, traveling around the globe even, is evidence enough that this is difficult, if not impossible, to contain.

The fields of organic farmers downwind from farmers using genetically engineered crops have been contaminated with these seeds through natural pollination methods. These farmers have been sued, their lives ruined by Monsanto for not having a "license" to grow Monsanto seeds. It truly is… well… just a mess. We trusted those whom we have elected to office and those whom they have appointed to governmental positions to protect us and our health. They have failed us and they have chosen instead to line their own pockets. Wendell Berry said it best: "A corporation, essentially, is a pile of money to which a number of persons have sold their moral allegiance." And might I add politicians?

There are those, like Jeffrey Smith, who have taken up the mantle and who are on the front lines fighting for us. There are those on the front lines who are fighting for food sovereignty and food freedom. There are farmers who are committed to growing only heirloom seeds using sustainable, organic, natural methods. There are people like me who are getting the word out to stop eating these Franken-foods.

Is it enough? It is certainly a start. Strides are being made. Money talks. Vote with your dollar. Support your local community and your local farmer; buy locally produced, organically grown food, meat, poultry, and raw dairy products.

I cannot urge you strongly enough, please stop eating foods that are genetically engineered, meat and poultry that are fed genetically engineered crops, and processed foods that are full of genetically modified ingredients. It is estimated that over 80% of commercially processed foods contain genetically modified ingredients. Please see the list of ingredients in the Appendix that are derived from genetically engineered crops. It is a very long list. These ingredients are in so-called "healthy" foods as well. Avoiding these organisms requires diligence.

If you have any health issues at all or if you want to avoid health issues in the future, you must first stop eating these ingredients.

As I sit here writing this section, I received a text from my mother with pictures of flowers that are blooming in her greenhouse; they are stunningly beautiful! God does not need our help! Yet, GMO can stand for "God Move Over" because that is what has happened. If you are a Christian, or even if you're not, you know that the way in which seeds were originally designed and the practices for planting, growing, and harvesting the food produced by those seeds that have been around since the beginning of time is already perfect. In His bountiful grace and mercy and goodness, He has given us what we need to nourish our bodies.

4 | What's for Dinner?

I dislike the thought that some animal has been made
miserable to feed me. If I am going to eat meat,
I want it to be from an animal that has lived a pleasant,
uncrowded life outdoors, on bountiful pasture,
with good water nearby and trees for shade.
Wendell Berry

A righteous man has a regard for the life of his beast,
but the compassion of the wicked is cruel.
Proverbs 12:10

I'm just going to be straight with you. This has been an incredibly hard chapter to write. I have had to view photos and videos of such horror and cruelty that it is almost impossible to rid these images from my mind. The tears flow freely. It is another reason why I write this book. It is another reason why I refuse to eat certain foods. I will do my best to describe some of these situations while avoiding the more graphic descriptions. Nonetheless, *Danger, Will Robinson! Danger!*

The Glory of God's Creation

We are created to honor our Creator and to bring Him glory in all that we do and in every aspect of life on this earth. Just as God created the seed that imparts life, so He has given us animals for food.

As Creator, God cares deeply for his His creation, and that includes animals, so much so that He bestowed the privilege of naming the animals to the first man, Adam; along with that privilege came the responsibility to care for those animals and to be good stewards of that gift to us. It matters to God that we treat these beings with dignity and not abuse them. It matters greatly. We are to be good shepherds and good stewards of the animals and the land and the resources which God has entrusted to us.

Regardless of your religious beliefs, the fair and good treatment of animals is just the morally right thing to do.

The Dignity of Animal Husbandry

If we look at animals, and particularly the animals we consume for food: cows, pigs, chicken, turkey, their natural habitat is grazing on wild grasses, foraging in vegetation hunting for protein, scratching the earth, in open fields and pastures, taking shelter from the sun under the shade of trees. This is where they thrive.

I think we can all agree that when you think of a cow, you think of them chewing their cud on the hills of rolling green pastures; they are herbivores after all, and grasses are their preferred food source. If you're from the south, you may be familiar with the idiom, "happier than a pig in mud." Despite the belief that pigs should be in pins of dirt and mud, that is not their true habitat. They are at their happiest when they, too, are strolling through deep vegetation, using their well-designed snout to root out the sources of rich protein hidden in the soil beneath the vegetation; they also like to nest there in that thick vegetation. In fact, contrary to popular belief, pigs in their natural habitat are very clean animals, building nests on hillsides so that the urine rolls downhill. They care for each other's piglets so that each sow can forage for food. Chickens are happiest when they are also roaming in open fields. Their pointed beaks and sharp talons allow them to scratch the earth and scratch through decaying manure to find sources of protein such as worms and larva, munching on grasshoppers, and the daily leftover vegetable scraps. While that may sound gross, it is how God designed them. And it is good.

The benefits of this type of farming are enormous. Cows are moved each day from one paddock or field, to another. The chickens are moved each day to the field vacated by the cows. This gives the land time to regenerate after grazing. The soil in fields like this is rich in many various types of vegetation; it is loose and not compacted; and rich in vital nutrients which are taken up by the plants the animals feed on. When farming is conducted using these methods, there is no need for hormones or antibiotics in the animals. There is no need for fertilizers or chemicals on the soil. This type of farming produces animals that are happy and healthy and it results in food that is nourishing for our bodies. It is effective and doable for farms of any size, large and small and it is surprisingly free of the foul odor typically associated with farms.

Think of the times you have been in the forest or a national park where the wild animals are protected and their numbers are high; does the forest smell foul? No. Nature, when left to do what nature does, takes care of itself. Confining pigs, cows, or chickens in a pin, even on a farm that is not an industrial concentrated feeding operation, is smelly business. If you've ever driven by a "chicken farm" where the chickens are housed entirely in long "chicken houses" you know the smell of which I speak; or if you have driven by a dairy farm where the farmer houses his cows in barns with concrete floors, you know the smell of which I speak. This does not occur when traditional farming methods that have been around for millennia are used.

Commonly, this type of historical farming is referred to as animal husbandry. The term husbandry implies and carries with it responsibility; a responsibility to care for the animals in a way that is humane and in providing an environment and food source that is natural to that animal. It carries with it a responsibility to protect the animal from harm, whether that is predators or shelter from severe weather. It is the act of lovingly caring for the animals that supply your family with wholesome food; treating them with dignity.

There are many reasons why this traditional type of farming and animal husbandry are beneficial and the mechanisms behind this are not only good for the animals, but also good for the earth in the way that it conserves or "sequesters" carbon rather than releasing it into the atmosphere; it doesn't rely on oil and fuel, chemical fertilizers, or tillage that destroys the soil. I'm not speaking of going back to the dark ages. Certainly there are new technologies that can be useful here, but the historical processes themselves, allowing nature to do what nature does, cannot be improved upon. As I have learned more about this topic, I find it quite fascinating and it reminds me that God's original creation was perfect and our "advances" are not necessarily a good thing when it comes to the planet and to the animals. Rather, just the opposite.[1]

While I would love to extrapolate at length the details of historical farming and its benefits for the animals and for the planet, it is beyond the purview of this chapter and it would, in fact, require an entire book to present this method in all its glory and others have done a much better job with that than I ever could. If this is something that interests you, I recommend the work of Joel Salatin. He is an expert in this area. My objective here is to illustrate to you that the way we do farming now, in a factory, is not natural, is not the best or most efficient way to farm, is certainly not in the best interests of the animals or the environment, and it is dreadfully far from producing nourishing food for our bodies, as you are about to learn.

IT'S WHAT'S FOR DINNER

Concentrated Animal Feeding Operations (CAFO)

Concentrated Animal Feeding Operations (CAFOs) are factory farms where animals are housed in factory-like buildings, crammed in cages, and sometimes tethered or chained. Yes, this is a contradiction in terms and morals. These animals are bred through industrial methods for the purpose of rapid growth and the production of large amounts of meat, milk, or eggs. Literally, thousands and thousands of animals are packed into conditions that are completely unnatural. These animals cannot breathe fresh air, forage, scratch the earth, or see the light of day. According to Daniel Imhoff, "Every year at least four domesticated animals are raised for every person on the planet. In the US alone nearly 10 billion domesticated livestock…are raised and slaughtered annually…"[2]

Following the Great Depression and World War II, there was concern among agriculture scientists that producing enough food for the country would be a problem, so they determined to figure out a way to increase production and increase our food supply. Also about this same time, new technologies were emerging in the area of agriculture and thus began the industrialization of traditional farming practices.[3]

There are some who contend that this progression from traditional animal husbandry to industrialized agriculture was a natural progression born out of necessity and not the result of cruel intentions. I am not convinced. Perhaps those early adopters to this new way of "farming" were simply following the herd (pun intended). Perhaps they really had no way to anticipate the consequences of sequestering thousands of animals whose natural habitat is wide open spaces into confined and cramped spaces would result in misbehavior by the animals caused by the anxiety and stress of confinement. Perhaps, but I'm not convinced they could not anticipate some of the fallout from these operations, particularly because these farmers would have been intimately acquainted with the habits and characteristics of these animals from years of caring for them in a natural environment.

There are many consequences produced by factory farms not only to the animals, but also to the environment. As well, much misinformation has been spread about these operations. Let's take a closer look.

Production-Specific Problems

Cows

Confining animals to small cages and enclosed spaces with no fresh air and no way to get out of their own muck, produces diseases which are directly a result of confinement. Beef cattle, for instance, are raised on grass, but for the last several months of their life, they are confined and fed a diet of genetically modified grain (which is not a natural food for cows), poultry and pig waste (protein), bone or meat meal (from chicken, pigs, and cows – though it is now illegal to feed cows to cows, it is suspected this still takes place since manufacturers of "protein" feeds will not disclose their ingredients), cement dust, and newspaper. The purpose of this is to fatten the cow at an incredible rate in preparation for slaughter. Most beef cattle, however, are raised in confinement and fed a diet of "forage" until the time of fattening with a high carbohydrate diet.

It generally takes several years for a grass-fed cow to grow large enough for slaughter. However, industrial beef cattle are brought to slaughter within 14-16 months. To hasten this fattening-up process, along with the unnatural diet, the animals are also given hormones. Because this is not a natural diet for these animals, they often develop liver abscesses, mad cow disease, and other illnesses; and since the animal protein they consume may come from infected animals, it is a vicious cycle of disease. To control the disease created by the horrendous diet, the animals, including those not currently suffering from disease, are given antibiotics.

Additionally, beef cattle are housed in dirt pins by the hundreds and spend their days standing in their own muck and that of other cows, often up to their knees. Muck, if you are not aware, is a slurry of animal waste, urine and feces, mixed with the dirt. When the cattle are sent for processing, they are doused with chemicals and irradiated to kill any pathogens present in the muck which is caked on their limbs and on their bodies.

There are times when this "cleansing" is not complete and an extremely virulent strain of *E.coli* enters the food supply, resulting in recalls, usually after sickness and sometimes deaths have occurred in the population.

For dairy cows, a normal life would be approximately 20 years. For factory-farmed dairy cows, their lifespan is typically 5 years. They, too, are injected with hormones, antibiotics, and fed a diet of corn, hay, cornstalk, silage, soybeans, and cottonseed (all genetically modified) all laced with chemical "buffers." The overload of carbohydrates causes severe bloating and gas. If the gas is not relieved, usually by crude means, the severe bloating pushes against the lungs and the cows suffocate and die. This unnatural diet also causes a build-up of acid in the stomachs of these cows as in the beef cattle, resulting in liver abscesses and painful conditions of the hooves. Mastitis, an inflammatory condition of the udder is another recurring problem. The pus created by the inflammation, aside from being extremely painful for the cows, ends up in the milk these cows produce.

These cows are confined in cramped quarters, never graze on grass, and only the "organic" cows are allowed time in the open air in dirt pins. When they calve, their babies are taken away, causing more stress, more inflammation, sicker cows who die an early death. Perhaps that is a blessing for these usually long-lived animals to not live in hell for 20 years.

Whether beef cattle or dairy cows, these animals are forced into environments that are artificial and unnatural. This produces a significant amount of stress on the animals which produces inflammation in their bodies which lowers their immune function which sets them up for disease along with the unnatural diet. Another perfect storm.

Swine

Pigs are social animals; in their natural environment, the sows take turns looking after the piglets so that they can forage and cover quite a lot of ground in one day. In factory farms, pigs are packed into the pig houses by the thousands in pens too small for them to turn around in, no straw to burrow down in, no sunlight, no fresh air, and floors with open slats for their animal waste to fall through. The air in a typical pighouse can exceed 90 degrees and exhaust fans must run continually, otherwise the air becomes toxic from the fumes of the waste products in the catch-pens beneath the "floors" which are also filled with spilled chemicals, antibiotics, afterbirth, piglets which have been accidentally crushed by their mothers, and anything else that can slip through those openings. If the fans break down for any length of time, the pigs begin to die for lack of oxygen. Once the waste catch-pens are full, the valves are opened and the waste is pumped into a retention pond.

The pigs in these CAFOs are artificially inseminated, the male piglets are killed, and the female piglets are quickly taken from the sow who has farrowed those piglets on the open-slatted floor of the "farrowing" area similar in size to the other pens; there is no room to turn around or move.

Confinement causes stress and anxiety and the pigs will eat and chew anything to relieve their anxiety. Their tails must be cut off, usually without any anesthetic, so the other pigs do not eat them. If there is a small wound, the pigs can become the victim of cannibalism from another pig. The stress of living in such conditions compromises their immune systems which generates a susceptibility to parasites, microbes, and other viral infections which requires the use of pesticides, antibiotics, and vaccines in large doses. When it is time for slaughter, the pigs are injected with as much medication as is necessary for them to be ambulatory so that they can make it to slaughter. Many pigs die on their way to the slaughterhouse in the semi-tractor trailers that transport them. To get an idea of just how many pigs are "grown" in factory farms, Jeff Tietz says it best:

> Smithfield Foods, the largest and most profitable pork processor in the world, killed 27 million hogs in 2007. That's a number worth considering. A slaughter-weight

hog is 50 pounds heavier than a person. The logistical challenges of processing that many pigs each year is roughly equivalent to butchering and boxing the entire human populations of New York, Los Angeles, Chicago, Houston, Philadelphia, Phoenix, San Antonio, San Diego, Dallas, San Jose, Detroit, Indianapolis, Jacksonville, San Francisco, Columbus, Austin, Memphis, Baltimore, Fort Worth, Charlotte, El Paso, Milwaukee, Seattle, Boston, Denver, Louisville, Washington DC, Nashville, Las Vega, Portland, Oklahoma City, and Tucson.[4]

That's just the largest producer, not all of them. I'm certain that number is much higher today; we can add a few more cities to that list. That is a lot of sick pigs and millions and millions of tons of toxic excrement.

Poultry

Chickens are also social animals. They like to scratch and peck and dustbathe and stretch their legs; but in chicken houses, they are packed in tightly. For broiler chickens, there are thousands and thousands of chickens crowded together, unable to move. As with cows and swine, they are pumped with hormones to increase their rate of growth. They grow so quickly and get so large that their legs are unable to keep pace and hold them up, so they lie around in their own excrement until the day of slaughter, if they survive that long. The air is toxic with high concentrations of ammonia. The sensitive end of the chicken's beak is seared off, without anesthetics, so that they do not peck each other as a result of stress and anxiety. They are injected with antibiotics to prevent disease such as the bird flu which can spread like wildfire through a hen house.

Egg laying hens are caged in "batteries" that are no larger than a piece of paper, stacked one upon the other, hundreds upon thousands of them in one hen house. They can't flap their wings or "nest" when it is time to lay eggs, an instinctual trait. They spend their entire life in a cage for the sole purpose of laying eggs. They, too, are given hormones and injected with antibiotics.

Have you seen the new commercial by poultry producers claiming to put oregano, a natural antibiotic, in their drinking water? Convincing? Makes for good marketing and good television, and while they may in fact do that, make no mistake, they are still using copious amounts of antibiotics.

Have you seen the labels for meat and eggs that these birds received a vegetarian diet? Chickens are first and foremost carnivores; they love grubs and worms and grasshoppers, all protein and while they do consume "vegetables," it is not their primary diet in nature. Clever marketing for the uninformed consumer.

What do you think of when you see the "cage-free" label? Chickens happily enjoying the sun and the grass and the places to nest away from prying eyes? That is not at all what that term means. It means what it says, the hens are not in cages; however, they are still in row upon row upon row of long "shelves" packed in tightly, wire-mesh bottoms so that their waste drops onto the heads of the hens below them. It simply means that they are not in a cage the size of an iPad; they are still confined in unsanitary conditions.

What do you think of when you see the "free-range" label? Chickens happily enjoying the sun and the grass and the places to nest away from prying eyes? No surprise that is not at all what that term means. It means that there is a dirt area outside of the chicken house enclosed with fencing and doors which open on to it; however, the majority of chickens will never reach that door because there are thousands of birds crammed in this space and it is impossible for them to make their way to the door if they are able to walk at all.

Egg hatcheries… almost too sad to describe. Thousands and thousands of eggs are hatched in incubators: large carts with about 10-12 bins in a warm closet. Once hatched, the baby chicks are thrown, along with the shells, onto a conveyor belt which separates the baby chicks from the shells. They travel through several conveyor belts and high speed shoots which literally propels them onto another conveyor belt until they are loaded and shipped to the factory farms. The baby chicks which are too weak and frail are dumped, along with the shells, into a large bin where an individual using a smashing tool, repeatedly beats them until they are crushed to death.

Can you imagine the sound of hundreds of thousands of baby chicks chirping for their mother? You see, baby chicks love to hide in her wings where they feel safe and protected unlike the cold industrial conveyor belts hurrying them to their destination in a cramped, over populated, chicken house where they will be injected with hormones to make them grow too fast and antibiotics to keep them "healthy" until their short days are up.

* * *

To be interested in food but not in
food production is clearly absurd.
Wendell Berry

While I have not specifically discussed farmed-fish here, know that the same problems exist in those operations as well: feeding with cornmeal – how is that a natural diet? - water pollution, confined environment, medications, disease. Wash. Rinse. Repeat.

Please do not be deceived by cunning advertising and marketing, whether it is for meat or poultry. The industry does not want you to know the truth about the living and health conditions of these animals; in a word, deplorable. They make it to slaughter only because they have been pumped full of medications. In other words, they are sick, all of them.

If an animal has a broken leg, for instance, it is usually left untreated; it is too costly and in the mind of the CAFO owner, unnecessary. They do not receive basic care beyond adulterated, unnatural to their diet, food, and water. All of the other necessities of life are taken from them: the ability to socialize in their natural environment, breathe fresh, clean air, the ability to eat a diet which is natural and nourishing. The absence of these things causes tremendous amounts of behavioral problems with these animals. They act out because they are imprisoned and they don't know why. It is completely unnatural to them. They are being poked and prodded and kicked and they have body parts cut off, in a confined space of concrete and dirt and they must breathe in toxic air, further destroying their immune system. It is a vicious cycle of abuse and sickness. It is inhumane what we are doing. If a person abuses a dog, they can be fined or jailed. How are farm animals any different?

Countering the Propaganda Machine

These concentrated animal feeding operations are industrial factories not farms. The animals are not "raised;" they are "grown" like a crop. Because these corporations are just that, large corporations, they have the ability to lobby heavily against regulations asserting that they are "agricultural farms" thereby bypassing industrial issues which are usually subject to regulation such as clean air and clean water. Because they are not legally considered an industrial enterprise, they are not liable for the damage they cause to the environment nor are they responsible to clean up the damage they cause to the environment without legal action being filed against them by local residents and entities.

Yet, these operations are, in fact, industrial, having no resemblance to farms. The scale of these operations, housing thousands and thousands of animals is well beyond the capacity of even a large farm. In fact, even the terminology they use to describe their operations have no resemblance to a farm: production units (animals), production facilities (buildings), processing facilities, etc. There is no pasture. There are no crops. Rather, concrete floors or open-slat floors, animals housed in indoor facilities with no room to move or turn around, and toxic air to breath. Not what I think when I think of farming.

While the cost of industrial food at the grocery store may be inexpensive, it is far from cheap. In fact, it is quite costly in a

number of ways. It is only because of enormous government subsidies that the food on your plate is "affordable." These subsidies
only go to the industrial factory feed operations rather than small
or even midsized real farms.

As mentioned earlier, CAFOs produce an exorbitant amount
of animal waste which must be disposed of. In a natural setting,
there is a symbiotic relationship between the animal (waste)
and the land, a beautiful dance, really. The animal feeds on the
foliage, fertilizes the land, which in turn grows more lush and
thus more nutritious foliage for the animal; an intricate ebb and
flow between the two. In a CAFO there is no such relationship.
According to the USDA, the animal waste produced by factory
farms is estimated to be about 500 million tons per year![5] This
is three times the amount of waste produced by humans which,
by law, must be treated; yet animal waste from CAFOs is not.
Rather, this waste is dumped into retention ponds where it seeps
into the ground water, surface water, and its toxic fumes pollute
the air in those communities. Additionally, it produces a legion
of flies that can trap people in their homes.

These toxic slurries contain hormones and antibiotics and all
manner of dangerous pathogens which can be inhaled or ingested
through drinking water, or contact with other water sources; this
is particularly dangerous for those living around these facilities.
Diseases attributable to these pathogens include:

- Anthrax
- Colibacilosis, Coliform mastitis-metris
- Leptospirosis
- Listerosis
- Salmonellosis
- Tetanus
- Histoplasmosis
- Ringworm

- Giardiasis

- Cryptosporidiosis

Symptoms associated with these include fever, vomiting, muscle aches, diarrhea, abdominal pain, nausea, skin rashes, weakness, and dehydration. Air quality is also an issue and emissions from CAFOs produce ammonia, hydrogen sulfide, and particulate matter, which cause chronic respiratory problems as well as skin rashes. Methane is a greenhouse gas and may contribute to changes in climate.[6]

When these facilities are located near rivers and streams and large bodies of water, during times of natural disaster or flooding, these retention ponds flood, wash into these bodies of water and millions upon millions of fish die. The waste is spread out over the land and everything is contaminated. It is an environmental nightmare and it requires costly legal action to hold these corporations responsible.

The health risks associated with CAFOs are profound and affect the workers as well as the consumer. Obviously, the workers are subject to all of the pathogens and emissions mentioned above. There have been reports of men who have fallen into hog CAFO retention ponds and died. It takes weeks to recover their bodies.

Antibiotic resistance has also been linked to the enormous amounts of antibiotics that are used in CAFOs each year. In 2011, in the United States, 29.9 million pounds of antibiotics were sold to CAFOs. That same year 7.7 million pounds were sold for human use.[7] That means that approximately 80% of the antibiotic use in the United States is used on animals in industrial factory farms! How does this translate into antibiotic resistance? When you consume these animals, you are also consuming antibiotics. When you consume these animals, you are also consuming the hormones and other medications and vaccines given them.

Put simply, consumers are eating sick and dying animals. Is it any wonder we are a nation of sick people?

Hazardous working environments for workers and property devaluation for communities surrounding these factories are two other deleterious effects of CAFOs. The loss of small farms has far-reaching effects as well. In short, CAFOs are environmental plights on the landscape, contaminating the water and the air, housing animals in warehouses where they are treated with horrific cruelty, and taking control of the food supply from local communities and putting it into the hands of a few large corporations.

*   *   *

The principle of confinement in so-called animal science is derived from the industrial version of efficiency. The designers of animal factories appear to have had in mind the example of concentration camps or prisons, the aim of which is to house and feed the greatest numbers in the smallest spaces at the least expense of money, labor, and attention. To subject innocent creatures to such treatment has long been recognized as heartless. Animal factories make an economic virtue of heartlessness toward domestic animals, to which we humans owe instead a large debt of respect and gratitude.
Wendell Berry

I'm not sure I've done justice to this vitally important issue here absent the more graphic, true-to-life descriptions, but I do hope that you realize the seriousness of this issue, not only for the animals, but also for those who consume these products.

It is easy to look the other way and hold a mindset that doesn't want to know the truth, but as Christians, we are called to a higher standard. We are called to stand up for those who can't stand for themselves. We are called to be good stewards of the land and of the animals which have been entrusted into our care. We are called to nourish our families, not poison them. I ask myself, how did this happen? How did we let this take place?

We have abdicated our responsibilities to those who do not have our best interests in mind. We have abdicated our responsibilities to the politicians we elect whom we think will represent our best interests. While there are some who do, I posit that most are swayed by the money they receive from the lobbyist of the mega-corporations and the power that affords them, rather than by the loyalty to their communities and the people who reside there. Because we have abdicated our responsibility, we also bear the blame. Ignorance is not bliss. The health of our families is too important to turn over to those whose main priority is money and not our health or the welfare of those animals.

I am happy to see that the tide is turning a little. Small farms are beginning to re-emerge. Local communities are coming together to provide clean and wholesome food for themselves. It is a move in the right direction, but there are still miles to go.

5 | Remember Nuremberg?

Primum non nocerum. First do no harm
Hippocrates

I find medicine is the best of all trades because whether
you do any good or not you still get your money.
Molière

Unless we put medical freedom into the constitution the time
will come when medicine will organize into an undercover
dictatorship and force people who wish doctors and treatment
of their own choice to submit to only what the dictating
outfit offers.
Dr. Benjamin Rush 1787
(Founding Father, signer of the
Declaration of Independence.)

The third leading cause of death in this country, behind heart disease and cancer, respectively, is iatrogenesis: the inadvertent or preventable induction of disease or complications by the medical treatment or procedures of a physician or surgeon; this includes the correct prescription for medications and taking them as prescribed. In other words, all those warnings about adverse reactions on the insert to a prescription and medical errors are the third leading cause of death in the United States each year claiming more than 250,000 lives.[1] One estimate puts this number at

780,000, which would make medical error the number one cause of death in the United States.[2]

My daddy was one of those people. I believe, after an informed analysis of his condition, that he was misdiagnosed with cancer and then prescribed chemotherapy at a very high dose which eventually took his life (This based on hours of research and conversations with his doctors wherein one stated he could find no evidence of cancer and believed he had another disease which is a "cousin" to that particular cancer). When he got to the point where it was obvious the chemo would kill him if he continued on that path, he stopped treatment stating that he would rather die of the disease than die from the treatment. It was horrific. The damage inflicted upon his body was irreparable, which eventually led to his death some years later. In the interim, he had no quality of life; it was taken from him. This man who was once fiercely independent, strong, and vital into his 70s, was reduced to a frail shell of a person, dependent on others for his care, no longer able to engage in the activities he once loved and enjoyed. For a man who took great pride in and who derived great pleasure from being the provider and the protector of the family, this was incredibly hard for him to bear.

He is just one of many.

Please hear me. I am not diametrically opposed to conventional, or allopathic, medicine. We have made tremendous strides, especially in emergency, trauma, and necessary surgical care. However, when it comes to chronic diseases, the medical establishment has failed us. I believe that most doctors do care and that they have a genuine desire to help patients, but they have high patient loads and limited time. Additionally, the primary focus of their training is in how to prescribe pharmaceutical drugs; they do not receive the necessary training to treat the whole person nor do they receive more than an hour or two of training in nutrition, if any at all. This leaves allopathic medicine at a great disadvantage. Yet, this is by design.

Charitable organizations, the pharmaceutical industry, and government entities influenced by these organizations, and the medical industry control the medical schools and what is taught and how care should be administered. Some of you may agree with me; others of you may think I am exaggerating, thinking it can't be as bad as all that. Let me explain how we arrived at this point with a little history lesson.

* * *

Disease is the warning, and therefore
the friend – not the enemy – of mankind.
George S. Weger, MD

I love history; it really is important and if we don't know our history, then we are destined to make the same mistakes over and over.

Hippocrates of Kros, (460-370 B.C.) is considered the "father of medicine." Today's Hippocratic Oath, which all doctors must recite, is a modern version of the oath Hippocrates formulated in ancient Greece. Some of his views on medicine are still adhered to today; some are not. He believed that the patient should be treated as a whole person. His first best quality as a person and as a physician was his integrity as evidenced by this oath (see the Appendix for a copy of the oath, both then and now.)

He based his medical philosophy around the Pythagorean Theorem, a concept in geometry, which states: the square of the hypotenuse of a right-angled triangle is equal to the sum of the squares of the two sides that make up its right angle. This concept is applied in nature as the basic elements of: water, earth, wind, and fire. In medicine, Hippocrates applied this same concept in the way that he approached healing. His theorized that the body is made up of four fluids or "humors": blood, phlegm, yellow bile, and black bile. He also translated this theory of elements to four conditions within the body: cold, hot, dry, moist. Hippocrates posited that the health of the human body was contingent upon the balance of these four elements and four humors, thus the theory of treating the person as a whole or what we refer to today as a holistic approach.[3]

Hippocrates believed that it was the physician's job to assist the body and the person to return to balance because medicine was an art and nature the artist, therefore, the physician and the patient worked together to heal the disease. He is quoted as saying, "Everyone has a doctor in him or her; we just have to help it in its work. The natural healing force within each one of us is the greatest force in getting well." The use of natural herbs, exercise, energy from the sun, food, and the axiom, "do no harm" were the foundations of his practice.

While some of the tenets of Hippocrates' practice and theories still remain, in the mid-19th century, the idea of "germ theory" became the predominant mode of thinking when it came to disease; this idea that bacteria is a bad thing and something to be eliminated at all costs. To be sure there were advancements in the understanding of immunology. The need for our bodies to produce immunities was discovered early in the 19th century when in Britain there was an outbreak of smallpox and only the milkmaids, who were exposed to "cowpox" when milking cows, were immune to the smallpox virus.[4]

Along came the French chemist, Louis Pasteur and his theory that all bacteria needed to be eliminated, the good and the bad; he did not distinguish between the two. As you know, the process of killing off all bacteria became known as pasteurization, especially as it relates to food and beverages. About this same time, another French scientist, Pierre Jacques Antoine Béchamp, discovered that it's not necessarily the bacteria that is inherently bad, but rather the "terrain" within which the bacteria is thriving. Béchamp believed, correctly, that bacteria don't just spontaneously appear, but rather that the environment in which these germs exist are what causes disease.[5]

To further Béchamp's theory, scientist Claude Bernard began to study why the germs act the way they do in certain environments. This work is what we know today as pH balance. Bernard was able to determine that the acidity or the alkalinity is what caused germs to go rouge or not; he coined the phrase, "The terrain is everything; the germ is nothing."[6] In other words, the germs are not harmful unless the environment is ripe for that to happen.

Needless to say, the discoveries by Béchamp and Bernard were diametrically opposed to the incomplete science of Pasteur. In fact, on his deathbed, Pasteur admitted that he had been incorrect and he agreed that the environment was the most important factor in promoting the growth of deadly bacteria.[7] To put it another way, the health of our internal bodies provides the right environment to either promote health or to promote disease. In short, the best defense against disease is a healthy immune system.

> Germs do not cause disease! ... As their [individuals]
> environment is, so will be the attraction for
> any specific micro-organism... The germ theory
> and vaccination are kept going by commercialism.
> Robert R. Gross, MD

In the 19th century and into the early 20th century, "regular" doctors used blood-letting by way of lancet, purgatives such as calomel (chloride of mercury), and arsenic to restore vigor. How any of these means and poisons could ever be considered a viable option that would restore vigor is beyond comprehension. These "remedies" were unpleasant and often lethal. Most people preferred the use of herbalists, eclectics, homeopaths, and osteopaths much to the chagrin of "regular" doctors. In fact, the upper class and the elite preferred homeopathy because it was effective, safe, and in no way unpleasant.[8]

Until the early 20th century when the tide began to shift, herbalism, eclectics and homeopathy were the predominant forms of medicine and in the United States there were many practitioners of these healing arts. While "regular" doctors often attended some type of university, the other "sectarian" practitioners were often apprenticed, though there were schools and lectures which they attended; and there were a lot of them, more than the "regular' doctors. These "regular" doctors saw this as a problem which needed a solution.[9]

What was the problem, specifically? Too many doctors diluted the money pool. In European countries like Germany, there was one doctor for every 2,000 people. In America, there was one doctor for every 568 people. "The chief complaints of the most prominent professional spokesmen by the end of the [19th] century were the 'surplus' of doctors, 'low' incomes, and the low social status of the profession."[10]

The American Medical Association (AMA) was formed by the different sects of "regular" doctors in 1847 to begin to mobilize and to discredit any practitioner not a "regular" doctor and it wanted to reduce the number of medical schools so as to reduce competition in order to reduce the number of doctors so that their incomes would increase along with their social status. The AMA is not a governmental agency, rather it is a labor union of physicians; they wear white collars instead of blue. The AMA was formed for the sole purpose of propelling doctors to the tops of the social and economic ladders.[11] In order to do this, they had a huge hurdle to overcome.

These "regular" doctors struck fear in the minds of the public and they were ridiculed for their crude means of "healing." The "quacks" as the AMA began to call began to call the herbalists, homeopaths, and osteopaths, on the other hand, had a strong base of support because their methods were safe, effective, and rarely resulted in death. Their methods promoted confidence rather than ridicule from the public. "They had a following, including many wealthy and influential people, who believed in their absolute effectiveness. Their practitioners were widely believed to be…as effective and certainly less dangerous than most regular doctors. And they did not demand a monopoly of practice…"[12]

> *We must admit that we have never fought the homeopath on matters of principle. We fought them because they came into our community and got the business.*
> Dr. J.N. McCormack, AMA 1903

Because homeopathy was so popular, these "regular" doctors decided to exclude them from their medical societies established through the AMA and to deny them hospital privileges. A massive campaign was underway to discredit them, and to deny them, as well as osteopaths and herbalist, from new licensing laws that were being introduced as a means of excluding those particular professions and in an attempt to elevate "scientific" medicine.[13] Despite these attacks and exclusions, homeopathy, osteopathy, and eclectic medicine remained very popular and the preferred options for the public.

Prior to 1910, there was a variety of medical education institutions: apprenticeships, proprietary schools, and university training. There were many different perspectives and the inquiry through science took many different forms which was considered normal and healthy for the profession. Also, it was "free-market" rather than controlled by a select few. "The ideological precedents for medicine was one that inherently disallowed the type of easily corruptible disease management techniques that we see so often today, and it's why medicine as a healing art flourished so beautifully during that time."[14] There was no one way and the idea of inquiry was available to anyone.

However, by 1910 the science of medicine, rather than the art of medicine, was being touted as the new direction for physicians and universities, offering full time teaching positions, rather than seeing patients. This was seen as a move up the ladder for many and with it came "prestige" and money. However, up and coming universities and laboratories were unable to sustain themselves, so they needed funding. Enter John D. Rockefeller of Standard Oil and the Carnegie Foundation.[15]

In 1910, John D. Rockefeller, Sr. (by way of J.D., Jr., and Senior's assistant, Frederick T. Gates) and the Carnegie Foundation commissioned what is known as the Flexner Report written by Abraham Flexner, a former teacher. Rockefeller and the Carnegies were interested in changing the path of medicine and the profession, so they commissioned Flexner to visit the medical schools across the country and make a recommendation;

this "recommendation" had already been pre-determined prior to Flexner undertaking his "study" of medical institutions.[16]

The pre-determined outcome of this report was that any medical school that taught therapies other than pharmaceuticals were pronounced "quacks" and "charlatans" and these medical schools were eventually closed. You see, Rockefeller needed the medical profession to prescribe more pharmaceutical drugs which are, in part, a derivative of petroleum, a/k/a Standard Oil of New Jersey. In order to keep the medical schools in check, the physicians' labor union, the AMA, was put in charge of who could enter medical school, which medical schools were following the standards of "conventional" medicine also known as prescription-based medicine, and which were not following this prescribed method or were also teaching homeopathy, osteopathy, eclectic, and herbal medicine. By the middle of the 20th century, all medical schools that did not adhere to the "conventional" pharmaceutical mode of medicine where shut down.

A Closer Look at the Flexner Report

In the early 20th Century, a group of men came together to form the project that became The Flexner Report and the beginning of our current medical system. The group formed in and through what was later to be named Johns Hopkins Medical School. The members included William Welch, the founding dean of Johns Hopkins; William Osler, the first chief of medicine; Frederick Gates, Rockefeller's assistant; and Abraham Flexner, a former school teacher (his brother, Simon, was a pharmacist).

Flexner, during his studies, had travelled to Britain, France, and Germany. He was particularly enamored with the German model of medical education and he was particularly enthralled with Theodore Billroth's text, *Medical Education in German Universities,* and used it as a basis of his analysis of American medical schools. This text contained many anti-Semitic references that are quite disturbing, as well as portraying the patient as nothing more than a means to an end, to serve the academic purposes of the faculty, "the patient was something to work on, interesting experimental material, but little more."[17] Yet, Flexner saw this text as "a work of enduring value."[18]

To be sure, the advancements in medicine and the knowledge that has been gained through scientific inquiry have contributed to a tremendous expansion in our understanding of the human body and of disease. Did these members of the Hopkins Circle and the Flexner report take humanity on a path that has led to overlook the reason for physicians in the first place? Has the human element been discarded for the sake of knowledge? Dr. Thomas Duffy found irony in the Teutonic or German influence on our current system in his analysis of the 100 year anniversary of the Flexner Report believing that the profession has lost its soul for the sake of knowledge, "It is the tale of Faust* and the irresistible allure of knowledge in exchange for one's soul. The Carnegie Foundation unwittingly recast Goethe's drama by selecting Flexner as the main character in their version of the play."[19]

Indeed, the desire for power and money and status led this group of men to sacrifice the art of medicine for the science of medicine. The desire for power and money and status blinded these men to the fact that the physician's primary role is that of a healer and the balance of patient care and science could, in fact, be mutually beneficial. The Flexner report sealed the fate of the American medical system to be forever tied to medical research. The German medical system relied on human experimentation.

The German Model

Rockefeller's Standard Oil of New Jersey owned a controlling interest in the German chemical company, IG Farben, the cartel which assisted Hitler in annihilating millions of people across Europe during World War II. In fact, IG Farben was the single

---

*   The legend of a German scholar who sold his soul to the devil in exchange for knowledge and power.

largest profiteer of Germany's attempted conquest during the war. Aside from being a chemical company, IG Farben was also a petro-chemical pharmaceutical company with its main plant at Auschwitz, Germany. This is the plant where they manufactured the poison gas Zyklon-B which was used for extermination in these camps. They used the camp at Auschwitz to test vaccines and other pharmaceuticals on the prisoners, most of whom died as a result of these experiments.

Rockefeller also supplied IG Farben with 500 tons of tetraethyl lead which the Germans needed for aviation fuel. The oil companies in the U.S. were the only ones with the technology to produce tetraethyl lead. One year later, he supplied the Germans with $20 million of tetraethyl lead. Later, during the war, Rockefeller would supply the Nazis with oil by diverting those shipments through Switzerland and would refuel German submarines in the Channel Islands and other areas for which he received a slap on the wrist from the U.S. War Department. Rockefeller used his influence to cancel bombing raids on the IG Farben complex and headquarters.[20]

During the Nuremberg War Criminal Tribunal in 1947, 24 of the board members of IG Farben were convicted of war crimes: mass murder, slavery, and other crimes against humanity, and were given very light sentences in prison. By 1951, all of those sentences were commuted and all of them continued to consult in German corporations. After the tribunal, IG Farben was dissolved into Bayer, BASF, and Hoechst (now Aventis). These companies are still in existence today and they are twenty times larger than their mother company IG Farben at its height in 1944.[21]

What is more disturbing is that for almost 30 years after World War II, these men convicted of crimes against humanity, filled the highest positions, chairmen of the board, at these pharmaceutical companies.

- Dr. Fritz ter Meer, who was directly involved in the development of Zyklon-B returned to work at Bayer where he remained chairman for 10 years.

- Carl Wurster, chairman of the board of BASF until 1974 was, during the war, on the board of IG Farben which manufactured the Zyklon-B gas

- Carl Winnacker, chairman of the board of Hoechst (Aventis) until the late 70's, was a member of the Sturm Abteilung (SA) and was a member of the board of IG Farben

- Curt Hansen, chairman of the board of Bayer until the late 70's, was co-organizer of the conquest of Europe in the department of "acquisition of raw materials." Under this leadership the IG Farben daughters, BASF, Bayer, and Hoechst, continued to support politicians representing their interests.

Others of the 24 convicted went on to hold position in sister chemical companies, banks, and universities; in other words, influential positions.[22]

The point of this bit of history? Those who wanted to change the state of medicine in the early to mid-20th century had ties to the medical system in Germany, the chemical cartels responsible for mass murder, and all that entailed. Rockefeller was in the oil business and he realized that he could use that oil to make patentable pharmaceuticals. Nature can't be patented, but drugs made with petro-chemicals can. A further point is that those who were convicted of war crimes and mass murder are the very men who headed up the drug companies producing the pharmaceuticals. Their interests were not in the health of the public.

Rockefeller and his various foundations, through extravagant donations, essentially controlled the medical system: what was taught; what wasn't taught; and who could participate; except they had one big hurdle to overcome. The people didn't want the "regular" doctors with their mercury and lancet and arsenic, they preferred the homeopaths, the osteopaths, and the herbalists. The AMA mounted a huge propaganda campaign which still churns today. They hired the best marketers who were fluent in persuasion and the use of classic techniques of appealing to one's emotions to sell their brand of medicine and convince the public that any form of medicine or healing outside of their "system" was quackery.[23]

The German Model in the 21st Century

Not much has changed. It is still happening today. What started out as a corrupt system has grown more and more corrupt. Daniel Weisberg, M.D. laments, "Built into the historic fabric of medical education is a tension between the values of scientific advancement and humanism in medicine. In the modern history of medicine, the latter struggles to find its place within a system built upon the German model of medical education and the research imperative."[24]

What is now referred to as "alternative" treatments was the gold standard for thousands of years. The problem with infectious diseases of the past was mostly eradicated with the advent of better sanitation and clean water. The illnesses and diseases we see today are a direct result of the toxins produced by an industrialized society, the heavy use of chemicals, the adulteration of our food supply, and the heavy use of synthetic, petro-chemical pharmaceuticals.

The pharmaceutical industry is not interested in your health. Your health is not in their bests interests. It is a for-profit industry with stock-holders who expect a significant return on their investments. We now have "diseases" that never existed before; they have been created by the industry to sell more drugs or they have hijacked things that happen naturally and are considered normal and turned them into a money-making machine. It's called "disease mongering" wherein drug companies try to convince healthy people they are sick and in need of drugs: restless leg syndrome, baldness, low testosterone (a natural occurrence that comes with aging), premenstrual dysphoric disorder, toenail fungus, social anxiety disorder, and the list goes on.[25] Most of these are natural occurrences and can be avoided or lessened with a proper diet.

In 1997, the FDA reversed its long-standing policy prohibiting drug companies from advertising to the public. This one act has opened up the flood gates and has sent patients clamoring to their doctors asking for specific medications. Dr. Jim Weber describes this phenomenon:

> Many times patients do come in asking us or telling us what it is they feel that they need. And oftentimes those medications come with a substantial side effect profile or the potential to create addiction. So as a physician, we are no longer really physicians, we are providers and our patients are really no longer patients, they are subjects enrolled in a third party healthcare system which has a legitimate stake in how we as physicians spend their money. The way we solve their problem in the short run is through the prescription and while that may be indeed a quick fix and a happy customer, we can't assume that our patients understand the concept of downright addiction. They understand that I give them a pill, they feel good, and their pain goes away without necessarily understanding the longer term repercussions. The central tenet of the physician-patient relationship is trust and if that trust is breached then we have a real problem on our hands and we are starting to see that now.[26]

The science of medicine has overtaken the art of medicine until the art of medicine is largely a thing of the past and replaced with drive through medicine fed by the hungry hounds of the pharmaceutical industry.

The amount of advertising by the pharmaceutical industry has increased exponentially since 1997, currently over $5.2 *billion* yearly.[27] In fact, the biggest recipient of this advertising money is the media.[28] Prescription drug advertising on television is now ubiquitous. Have you noticed that news segments are bracketed by commercials for prescription medications with the exhortation to "ask your doctor if this drug is right for you?" Prescription drug costs for 2015 were an exorbitant $425 *billion* and it is expected to reach $610-$640 *billion* by 2020.[29] Seven out of ten people in the U.S. are on at least one prescription medication and half of the population is on two medications and 20% of Americans are on at least five medications.[30] The United States represents 5% of the world's population, but it consumes more than 50% of the world's pharmaceuticals and 80% of the world's narcotics. Three times as many people die each year from prescription medication than die from heroin, cocaine, and methamphetamine combined.[31]

An additional problem with this advertising, especially as it relates to the media, is that the pharmaceutical industry controls what the media reports or doesn't report. According to John Abramson, M.D., in his book *Overdosed America*:

> The medical industry has finely honed its ability to mold public knowledge about the best medical care – slanting our beliefs in favor of the most profitable medical therapies . . . More insidious – and, for that reason, potentially more influential – are the public relations campaigns that translate into seemingly unbiased news stories and nonprofit public awareness campaigns.[32]

It is one way of suppressing information on natural therapies, the importance of vitamins and minerals in health, and promoting treatments and regimens that benefit the industry. Rather, it promotes consumption as a way of life and that happiness and health can only be attained through the use of prescriptions. Cue the happy people smiling as they walk with their loved ones, or one of many other such "settings" that depict all is well with the world when you take such and such prescription. In other words, as has been happening since the beginning of the modern medical era, the pharmaceutical industry controls the flow of information with propaganda through media channels.

Ignorance and arrogance make a bad combination,
and "modern" medicine has been guilty of both for decades.
The news media have been their willing accomplices. The
misinformation they spew to this day is fraught with
fabricated frights of natural therapies, while in the same
breath they spew forth the wonders of pharmaceutical drugs.
Andrew Saul

As with advertising and the media, so it is with politicians and the passage of laws and regulations. The medical industry – pharmaceutical companies, insurance companies, health professionals, hospitals, and nursing homes – contributed $160 *million* to the political campaigns for the 115th Congress. This includes the cycle of 2012-2016 for Senators and the 2016 cycle for members of the House. The highest ranking senators received upwards of $2 million and some more than $3 million in campaign contributions.[33] There are more pharmaceutical industry lobbyists (at least 625) than there are members of Congress. According to the Center for Public Integrity, the pharmaceutical industry and allied advocates spent more than $880 *million* on lobbying and political contributions at the state and federal level over the past decade.[34] How can we expect our elected representatives to keep the interests of their constituents as top priority? The only thing they need more than money is your vote. Both sides of the isle are guilty.

During the Bush 43 administration, Medicare Part D was introduced and passed through Congress. ALL of the sponsoring senators and congressmen had ties/relationships to the pharmaceutical industry and/or they had received hundreds of thousands of dollars from the industry through campaign donations or through lobbyists. The result of this bill for the pharmaceutical industry meant that they realized an $8 *billion* increase in profits. In 2003, the industry spent $116 million lobbying for Medicare

Part D. This bill gave the pharmaceutical industry the ability to name its price for drugs, get that price, and have the government, a/k/a, you and me the taxpayer, foot the bill without any negotiation of price.[35]

Prior to this bill passing, Jim Nicholson, then chairman of the RNC, wrote a letter to Charles Heimbold, chairman and CEO of Bristol-Myers Squibb wherein he expressed a desire to form a coalition with the pharmaceutical industry, "We must keep the lines of communication open if we want to continue passing legislation that will benefit your industry."[36]

I am in no way finding fault with Medicare; not at all. What I am demonstrating is that this bill, as an example, was created by the pharmaceutical industry for the pharmaceutical industry with the assistance of members of Congress.[37] The amount of fraud, abuse, and over-billing within Medicare is, quite frankly, out of hand and Congress refuses to deal with the issue.[38] I wonder why that is.

Research, Bought and Paid For

In 1992, Congress passed the Prescription Drug User Fee Act (PDUFA) wherein drug companies agreed to a "user fee" of $300,000 for each new application they submitted for drug approval. Their complaint had been that the approval process time, an average of 20 months, was too long. They lobbied Congress for this new Act and agreed to this fee so that the FDA's Center for Drug Evaluation and Research could fund more employees to expedite the approval process. In the first four years following the passage of the PDUFA, the length of time for drug approval dropped from 20 months to six months. This resulted in double the number of new drugs on the market.[39] Keep in mind that the FDA's primary role is to protect the public. Can an organization, half of whose budget comes from the pharmaceutical industry, act in a way that is unbiased?

Following this new approval process, the number of drugs being withdrawn from the market because of safety concerns rose

dramatically from 1.6% to 5.3% as a result of inadequate testing and evaluation. The FDA frequently disregards the warnings
of its specialists,[40] just as they did with genetically engineered
organisms.

At one time, the prestigious medical journals such as *Journal
of the American Medical Association,* the *New England Journal of
Medicine,* and *The Lancet* were a trusted source of the newest
and latest in medical research and study. However, in 2001, the
editors of twelve of these journals issued a statement that "told
of 'draconian' terms being imposed on medical researchers by
corporate sponsors. And it warned that the 'precious objectivity'
of the clinical studies that were being published in their journals
was being threatened by the transformation of clinical research
into a commercial activity."[41]

Indeed, this warning came to pass. Today, the pharmaceutical
and biotech industries fund their own studies. To be sure, these
studies are designed with a predetermined conclusion in mind
and are thus executed to reach this predetermined conclusion.
As with the "bad science" surrounding genetically engineered
organisms, so it is with medical trials and studies. The pharmaceutical industry can set their own rules and since the academic
institutions performing these studies are in competition with
other institutions for these monies, the pressure is on to com-
promise principles and morals and previous standards. "They are
seduced by industry funding, and frightened that if they don't go
along with these gag orders, the money will go to less rigorous
institutions. It's a race to the ethical bottom."[42] The scientific
integrity which was once the crowning jewel of these prestigious
institutions has bowed down to the highest bidder.

In fact, the majority of science is "bogus" according to
Richard Harris and cannot be replicated.[43] Some of the problems
with these studies:[44]

- Manipulating the dosing; using the wrong or incorrect
  placebos
- Studying the wrong patients

- The time frame of the studies are too short
- Revealing only the data that supports their intended goal
- Using ghostwriters – the company writes the science and pays an academic to sign the report

Tenure and promotions depend on research being picked up by the major journals and research dollars are at stake; add to that the research that is bought and paid for already and it is difficult to trust any of the research that is not completely independent.

And what about the doctors? While I do believe that most of them sincerely care about their patients, they are also uninformed or at best misinformed. The foundations which support medical education are also the foundations who advocate pharmaceutical-based medicine. The medical journals, as has been established, are filled with science that has been paid for by the industry. The pharmaceutical reps who visit their offices are certainly biased. The medical conferences they attend are also sponsored by the pharmaceutical and insurance industries.[45]

There are revolving doors between governmental agencies, FDA, NIH, and the CDC with physicians and scientists going from governmental agencies to pharmaceutical agencies and back again; as with those influencing policy regarding genetically engineered organisms, the lines are blurred and the influence by these billion dollar industries take precedence over public health and safety which is why the third leading cause of death in this country is at the hands of the pharmaceutical industry and the medical system.

Vaccines

I would be remiss if I did not include here a discussion on vaccination. I believe there needs to be a conversation and a closer examination of the ingredients in vaccines, their safety, and the necessity of vaccines. They are not all necessary. In many instances, creating a healthy immune system is all that is required.

There are some "diseases" such as measles, which are relatively harmless and studies have shown that having had the measles is a protection against cancer later in life.[46]

Newborn babies, even when the mother tests negative for Hepatitis B, are given the Hepatitis B vaccine. Why?! Hepatitis B is a sexually transmitted disease. Why would a baby only a few hours old whose mother is negative for Hepatitis B, need that vaccine? It is pure insanity; and that is just the beginning.

There is much harm that is happening to our children as a result of the vaccine schedule. By the time an infant is one year old, he has received 26 vaccines! Almost always, the shots contain 8, 10, or 13 different vaccines in one shot at one time. The number of vaccines administered to children from birth to age 17 has increased from 7 in 1950 to 74 in 2017. That represents a 414% increase in the number of vaccines.[47]

- In 1950, there were 7 childhood vaccines typically given by the time a child was 6 years of age.

- In 1983, there were 10 recommended vaccines by the age of 6 years old (24 doses, 7 injections, 4 oral doses for polio).

- In 2010, the CDC vaccine schedule totaled 68 doses with more than half given by the time a child was only a year and a half old.

- In 2017, the schedule has increased to 74 doses by age 17 with 53 injections and 3 oral doses of rotavirus.[48]

This escalation in dosing has created an epidemic of chronic illnesses in children; there is a direct correlation between the increase in the number of vaccines and the rise in childhood illness:

- 1 in 3 children are overweight
- 1 in 6 children have learning disabilities

- 1 in 9 children have asthma
- 1 in 20 children under the age of 5 have seizures
- 1 in 50 children have autism (this is expected to be 1 in 2 by 2030)
- 1 in 400 children have diabetes

Two month old babies receive a shot containing as few as 8 vaccines and as many as 13 vaccines at one time. Even though the vaccine schedule recommended by the CDC of 49 doses of 14 vaccines administered by the age of 6 is mandated in many states, the safety has not been tested according to the Institute of Medicine of the National Academy of Sciences:

> First, the concept of the immunization "schedule" is not well developed in the scientific literature. Most vaccine research focuses on the health outcomes associated with single immunizations or combinations of vaccines administered at a single visit. Even though each new vaccine is evaluated in the context of the overall immunization schedule that existed at the time of review, individual elements of the schedule are not evaluated once it is adjusted to accommodate a new vaccine. Key elements of the immunization schedule—for example, the number, frequency, timing, order, and age at the time of administration of vaccines—have not been systematically examined in research studies.[49]

As with other pharmaceuticals and genetically engineered crops, vaccine safety studies are either non-existent, or they suffer from the same issues of bad science as I have explained earlier. In the words of Dr. Tetyana Obukhanych, "I never imagined myself in this position, least so in the very beginning of my Ph.D. research training in immunology. In fact, at that time, I was very enthusiastic about the concept of vaccination, just like any typical immunologist. However, after years of doing research in immunology, observing scientific activities of my superiors, and analyzing vaccine issues, I realized that vaccination is one of the most deceptive inventions the science could ever convince the world to accept."[50]

To add insult to injury, in 1986 the vaccine industry went before Congress and told them that they were going to stop making vaccines because there were too many suits claiming vaccine injury and it was no longer profitable for them to make vaccines. This meant that in the event of an epidemic or an act of bioterrorism there would be no way of making vaccines in those emergencies; so in order for the vaccine industry to continue making vaccines, they were granted immunity from any liability associated with adverse effects, injury, or death as a result of the vaccines when Congress passed the National Childhood Vaccine Injury Act of 1986. No longer could a parent or guardian sue the vaccine maker in civil court; instead there is a separate federal court system specifically for vaccine injury. The law acknowledged that vaccine injury exists and there is an excise tax of $.75 per vaccine which goes into the coffer for this court to pay to vaccine injured individuals. As of 2012, the court had paid out over $3 *billion* in damages to children injured by vaccines.[51]

This law effectively relieves vaccine manufacturers from any liability whatsoever. What other industry is allowed to operate exempt from liability? In 1986, the number of vaccines a child received was 10; by 2013, that number had risen to 69. What incentive do they have to test for safety and effectiveness? What incentive do they have for quality control? They are free to use any ingredients they wish and the list is long.

Aside from the attenuated version of the virus or bacteria, the ingredients in vaccines are quite toxic and at levels many times higher than is considered safe by the FDA and EPA. Here are just a few:

- Thimerosal (50% ethylmercury) (neurotoxin) (in childhood vaccines and the flu shot) (more toxic than the methylmercury highly regulated in fish)

- Aluminum (can create food allergies and auto-immunity)
- Formaldehyde
- Antibiotics (neomycin)
- Chicken embryos
- Monkey kidney cells
- Aborted fetal tissue
- Triton-100 (surfactant found in industrial cleaners, household cleaners, paint, pesticides)
- Polysorbate-80 (used to open blood-brain barrier when giving chemo for brain tumor patients; binds tightly to aluminum, which binds tightly with bacteria and viruses, and carries it all into the brain; also opens tight junctions in the gut lining)
- Glyphosate (opens blood-brain barrier)
- Ethylene glycol (basically anti-freeze)
- Phenols[52]

This list is horrifying! And this is not the entire list. It should strike terror in the heart of any parent. This is what is being injected into our children and into adults, and especially the elderly.

The level of aluminum and mercury in the vaccines is much higher than the safe levels established by the FDA and the EPA. For instance:[53]

- The amount of aluminum in the seven doses give at the two-month baby check-up is 1,000 mcg
- The maximum allowable aluminum per day for intravenous parental feeding for healthy baby of eight pounds is 18.16 mcg
- The amount of aluminum received by fully vaccinated eighteen-month old baby is 5,000 mcg

- There are zero studies proving the safety of injecting aluminum into human infacts.

- The amount of mercury in liquid waste considered toxic by the EPA is 200 ppb

- The amount of mercury in large predator fish is 700 ppb

- The amount of mercury in "thimerosal-free" vaccines is 2,000 ppb

- The amount of mercury in some single-dose and some infant flu shots is 25,000 ppb

- The amount of mercury in multi-dose flu vaccines given to pregnant women is 50,000 ppb

- The amount of mercury needed to kill human neuro-blastoma cells is 0.5 ppb

Mercury is listed by the CDC as the third most toxic substance known, yet our children are being injected with this toxin many times over.[54]

According to Robert F. Kennedy, Jr., founder of the World Mercury Project, there are almost 500 studies on mercury and virtually all found that thimerosal is a neurotoxin. It is the most neurotoxic element in the universe that we know of that is not radioactive; it causes damage to other organs in the body; and it is reactive to human tissue. There are no studies showing that mercury is safe; however, there are 81 studies that link mercury toxicity to autism.[55]

Mercury is considered a hazardous waste, meaning that if the vial is dropped in the doctor's office everyone must evacuate the building and the hazmat team must be called in to clean it up, yet they inject the element into our children. Mercury is in the flu shot which is recommended for pregnant women and can cross over into the placenta and into the growing fetus.[56]

An additional problem is the administration of Tylenol to reduce fever following vaccination. Acetaminophen blocks the liver's production of glutathione which is an antioxidant that assists the body in detoxification of toxins, i.e., mercury and aluminum. In other words, the use of Tylenol or acetaminophen all but ensures that the baby's body will not expel the toxins. This is especially harmful for males because the negative effects of Tylenol are increased in the presence of testosterone.[57] This may explain why more males have autism than females.

Babies are not born with a mature and fully functioning immune system; as a result, most countries do not vaccinate until two years of age.[58] According to a 2011 independent study by Human and Experimental Toxicology, the United States, which mandates 26 vaccines before the age of one, has the highest infant mortality rate of any industrialized nation, coming in dead last of 34 countries, despite spending more than any of the other 33 countries on healthcare. "These findings demonstrate a counter-intuitive relationship: *nations that require more vaccine doses tend to have higher infant mortality rates*" (emphasis theirs).[59] The authors of the study further state that the situation appears to be worsening.[60]

Vaccine Paradox

Many of the vaccines administered are not necessary, for a number of reasons. The rotavirus vaccine, for example, is completely unnecessary. The worst possible thing that can happen is that the child becomes dehydrated and we are more than adequately equipped in this country to deal with dehydration, so the need for a vaccine is illogical. My youngest child had rotavirus when he was a baby and I admit it was not fun, but the worst of it lasted less than 24 hours. A serious problem with this vaccine is that it has introduced retro-viruses (from animal cells) into the human genome. These retro viruses perform what is referred to as "reverse transcriptase activity" which writes backwards the RNA into DNA and inserts itself into the human DNA where it remains for generations. Put simply, this vaccine has introduced into the human population retro viruses that have not been there before and that are responsible for many types of cancer.[61]

Additionally, the vaccine for rotavirus has created a new, more viral strain, norovirus, which is much worse than the rotavirus. This is happening with many of the viruses and bacterial vaccines; it is akin to antibiotic resistance in that these viruses and bacteria mutate into new, stronger strains than the one being vaccinated against. While bacterial infections such as meningitis can be very serious, the vaccine has compounded the situation. Whereas, viral infections such as chickenpox and measles are relatively harmless and infer life-time immunity, instill a robust immune system, and offer protection from other illness later in life such as cancer. In many instances, the vaccine facilitates or causes the spread of these diseases.[62]

Infants have an immature immune system and their bodies are not capable of handling many of these viruses and bacteria; however, if the mother is immune, she passes that protection on to her baby. The problem arises when the mother has been vaccinated which means that she has very low levels of antibodies, if any, to pass on to the child. According to Dr. Tetyana Obukhanych, "Many viral diseases are sometimes referred to as childhood diseases, because prior to the routine childhood vaccination, these diseases occurred mainly in children. Infants were protected from these diseases by maternal immunity, whereas adults were protected by their own life-long immunity, which they had acquired in childhood. The use of vaccines changed this pattern."[63]

Measles in infancy, for example, can put the baby at risk for measles infection of the brain called *subacute sclerosing panencephalitis* (SSPE). The rate of SSPE in the 1960s and 1970s was 8.5 cases of SSPE in 1,000,000 cases of measles. In the early 1990s the rate of SSPE was much higher at 12 cases per 55,622 cases of measles. This massive increase in the incidence of SSPE in the 1990s is directly related to the introduction of the measles vaccine in the 1960s which resulted in the absence of maternal immunity related to vaccination.[64] Per Dr. Obukhanych:

> Disrupting the natural cycle of the mother-infant immunity transfer is an unintended consequence of prolonged

vaccination campaigns. The risk of contracting the disease is simply pushed from childhood into adulthood, while vulnerable infants are left without any protection whatsoever. The vaccine paradox is that vaccines reduce the overall incidence of childhood diseases, yet make them infinitely more dangerous for the next generation of babies.[65]

Vaccines create more problems than they solve.

There is a new etymological pilot study titled "Pilot comparative study on the health of vaccinated and unvaccinated 6- to 12- year-old U.S. children" which revealed the following results for vaccinated children:

- A 4.2-fold increase in Autism Spectrum Disorder (ASD) and Attention Deficit Hyperactivity Disorder (ADHD)
- 5.2-fold increase in Learning Disability
- 3.7-fold increase in Neurodevelopment disorders (NDD) of any type
- Preterm birth and vaccine was associated with 6.6-fold increased odds of NDD.

The study also concluded that the children who received vaccinations were significantly more likely to suffer with immune-related disorders and the risk of allergic rhinitis (hay fever) was over 30 times higher along with a 3.9-fold increased risk of other allergies and a 2.9-fold increase risk of eczema.[66]

It bears repeating, the vaccine industry is free from liability for injury, and therefore, have no incentive to test for safety. According to the Vaccine Adverse Events Reporting System (VAERS), there were 45,742 reported events in 2016. In the first 75 days of 2017, there were 5,244 reported events with many more going unreported because parents and doctors consider certain symptoms coincidence, including skin rashes, high fever, seizures, swelling, and SIDS. In 2016, there were 1,120 claims filed with the federal vaccine injury court and in the first quarter of 2017, there have been 633 claims filed.[67] Vaccine safety, the number of vaccines administered at a time, and the number of vaccines in total, merit further study.

There is under development a new vaccine that would rewrite itself into your DNA called vectored immunoprophylaxis.[68] It is akin to the genetically engineered organisms in crops. Genetically modify humans. What could possibly go wrong?! Just as with GE crops and the unintended consequences of splicing the gene of another species into a plant, there will be unintended consequences. But that aside, the moral and ethical implications of this defy logic. Or perhaps we have lost our moral compass altogether. Is it not enough that they have played God with our food, now they want to inject us with a "vaccine" that will rewrite the human genome? And this at the same time there is a push to federally mandate everyone be vaccinated. What other genes will they include in those "vaccines?" Something is rotten in Denmark.

Collusion and Deception

As with the biotech industry, so it is with the pharmaceutical industry. The lines are blurred between the industry and the governmental agencies assigned to oversee it. Robert F. Kennedy, Jr., who heads up the World Mercury Project, questioned officials with the federal agencies, specifically Paul Offit, a former member of the CDC Advisory Committee on Immunization Practices and holder of a patent for the rotavirus, and Cathleen Straten of the CDC, had this to say: "When I started drilling down on them on the science [about mercury in vaccines] it was clear that not only was the science they were citing was bogus, but that they knew it was weak and they were unwilling to defend it ... it is manipulated science and it is criminal."[69]

The science isn't the only thing being manipulated or bought. Vaccines are good for business. The pharmaceutical industry is a trillion-dollar a year industry with vaccine sales annually accounting for $25 billion. Since the CDC mandates vaccines, the industry saves billions in advertising. There are 271 new vaccines in development; this could net the pharmaceutical industry $100 billion by 2025. Dr. Paul Offit, a board member of Every Child by Two, said "he believes children can take as many as 10,000 vaccines."[70] Insanity! Or is it corruption?

The corruption at the CDC runs deep and wide and the health of America's public is not their sole priority, or even a priority at all. "Four scathing federal studies, including two by Congress, one by the US Senate, and one by the HHS Inspector General, paints the CDC as a cesspool of corruption, mismanagement, and dysfunction with alarming conflicts of interest suborning its research, regulatory, and policymaking functions."[71] Not surprisingly, the rules of the CDC allow those with ties to the vaccine industry to serve on advisory boards. Dr. Offit, who sold his patent for the rotavirus vaccine for $182 million, was allowed to serve on the board, the same board that added the rotavirus to the CDC vaccine schedule, allowing him to sell his vaccine to the highest bidder, Merck. He told *Newsweek* "It was like winning the lottery!"[72] These federal studies found that the CDC certified financial disclosures even though they contained omissions and it found that 64% of the members of the committee had conflicts of interest and the CDC looked the other way.

Additionally, the research department of the CDC responsible for testing and safety is not without corruption as well. In 2014, Dr. William Thompson, a 17 year veteran of the CDC evoked "whistle-blower" status and handed over volumes of files to Congress of a principle study on thimerosal in the MMR vaccine which found a causative link between the vaccine and the incidence of brain injury and autism. Dr. Thompson had been ordered to manipulate the data and to lie and to destroy the files.[73] The movie *Vaxxed: From Cover-up to Catastrophe* documents this cover-up in startling detail.

The Healthy People 2020 initiative contains 400 goals and 1200 objectives. One goal is to take away your right to refuse vaccination.[74] In 2010, Bill Gates and the Gates Foundation declared this to be "The Decade of Vaccines" funding the initiative with $10 million. He has his hands in other global initiatives as well. Make no mistake, Bill Gates is not interested in the health of your children or the world's children. In a TedTalk that he gave in February, 2010 on climate change, he posits that the population of the planet is one of the variables responsible for rising CO_2 levels. This is how he explained his solution to this problem as regards decreasing the population: "If we do a really great job on new vaccines, healthcare, reproductive health services, we could lower that [the world population] by perhaps 10 or 15 percent."[75] In other words, kill the babies before they are born or with vaccines after they are born or through the healthcare system. He didn't skip a beat. I was stunned.

Censorship and Indifference

As I have mentioned earlier, the pharmaceutical industry, through its billions of advertising dollars, controls the news outlets, which are now the channel for the propaganda platforms of the industry. The spokespeople for the industry, like Dr. Offit, spread the industry lies, while the news outlets censor any criticism or other voices questioning the vaccine industry, declaring them all "anti-science" and much worse. I ask you, have you heard of the information here, in this chapter, and previous chapters, through mainstream media channels? I had not, nor have you. The movie *Vaxxed: From Cover-up to Catastrophe* was scheduled to premiere at the Tribeca Film Festival, but pulled at the last minute. Why?

The pharmaceutical industry is not interested in your health; they have no incentive in your being well and healthy. Think about it. They rely on your need for medications to stay in business. If you are well, have a strong immune system as a result of eating whole foods free of chemicals and genetically engineered organism, hormones and antibiotics, and use natural therapies, which aren't patentable, to support your immune system, then a huge portion of their revenues will be lost. They are only interested in generating a steady stream of profit.

The pharmaceutical industry has gone and does go to great lengths to suppress any knowledge available to the consumer about natural therapies. The very science that they used in the early 20th century to quash legitimate medical schools is the very science that they now try to suppress which clearly demonstrates that nutritional deficiencies are a big cause of disease, both physical and cognitive, the remedy for which is nutrient dense whole foods, herbs, and other natural therapies. They have resorted to attempting to discredit scientists and physicians who speak out in opposition to their propaganda.

In Chapter 2, I listed many different "diseases" that now afflict the population; these are all modern diseases which have occurred due to the industrial revolution. So whether it be chronic diseases, cancer, vaccine injury, behavioral, cognitive, the pharmaceutical industry wants you to take a pill or have surgery or get a vaccine, not because they are interested in your health, but because they are interested in the health of their bottom line. I have provided Resources in the back of this book so that you can begin your own journey and your own search for truth, because, YES, there are cures for cancer and YES, you can restore your physical and cognitive health without the use of petro-chemicals!

You have a choice. Make informed decisions. Do the research. Forced vaccinations? Yes, they care coming down the pike if we do not stand up now. Remember Nuremberg? This choice to refuse a vaccine or to refuse chemotherapy or other treatments is solely your right, as an individual and as a parent. No one has the right to force this on you or your children. It is the most basic and sacred of all human rights: the choice over your own body. Now, I am not talking about abortion here because that involves the life of another human being and a discussion which is beyond the scope of this text. I am referring to the right to decide for yourself or your children what you will or will not allow in terms of your body.

I am reminded of Elie Wiesel, a survivor of the concentration camps of World War II, and his book *Night*. He passed away in 2016. I believe that if he were here today and if he were aware of these truths, he would be standing alongside Robert F. Kennedy, Jr., and the other warriors for food safety and health, demanding answers and demanding that the truth be made known, because what we are experiencing now is not so dissimilar from what he experienced in those camps. The only difference is that we are not in an actual camp; rather we are being deceived by the very people who have been assigned to protect us and by those who, like IG Farben, are experimenting on our children and on our population. We have been lulled into complacency and indifference.

I leave you with three profound quotes from Elie Wiesel to ponder. (See also an excerpt from his speech, "Perils of Indifference," in the Appendix).

Indifference is the sign of sickness,
a sickness of the soul more contagious than any other.

To remain silent and indifferent is the greatest sin of all.

The opposite of love is not hate, it is indifference.

May we be the Dietrich Bonhoeffers of our day.

6

Toxic Overload

*The consideration of man's body has not changed to
meet the new conditions of this artificial environment
that has replaced his natural one. The result is that of
perceptual discord between man and his environment.
The effect of this discord is a general deterioration of
man's body, the symptoms of which are termed disease.*
Professor Hilton Hotema

One of the things I remember about studying biology in college
was the sheer amazement at the processes that occur at the cellular level in the body. I find it astonishing and miraculous that
so much can go on in something too small for the human eye to
see. Life happens there.

God has designed our bodies so beautifully with an innate
ability to heal itself. Our bodies instinctually lean toward health.
Did you know that? Your body is designed to fight disease and
restore health. There are processes in place within our bodies that
create and maintain homeostasis, or balance, which are designed
to keep our bodies operating optimally. I never cease to marvel at
this fact. I also take comfort in this fact. It gives me hope.

It has become harder and harder for our bodies to maintain
homeostasis. We are bombarded every day with a plethora of
heavy metals and chemicals from every direction:

- Food
- Water
- Air
- Cosmetics
- Plastics
- Cleaning products
- Scented candles and air fresheners
- Cookware
- Personal hygiene products
- Industrial pollutants
- Preservatives
- Flame retardants
- Pesticides and herbicides
- Mold

They are ubiquitous and almost impossible to escape. Avoiding them takes diligence.

The quality of your life is dependent upon the quality
of the life of your cells. If the bloodstream is filled with
waste products, the resulting environment does not promote
a strong, vibrant, healthy cell life-nor a biochemistry capable
of creating a balanced emotional life for an individual.
Tony Robbins

The EPA, pursuant to the Toxic Substances Control Act (TSCA), maintains an inventory of confidential and non-confidential chemicals that are registered. Currently, there are more than 85,500 non-confidential registered chemicals in use in the United States today. There is another list, one that is confidential, that the public is not allowed to see because they are considered trade secrets. We do not know the companies, the names of these chemicals, how and where they are being used, but we do know that there are many chemicals, in addition to the 85,500, that are in use. The types of chemicals on these lists include:

- Organics
- Inorganics
- Polymers,
- Chemical substances of unknown or variable composition, complex reaction products, and biological materials (UVCBs)

This list of over 85,500 does <u>not</u> include those chemicals not regulated under the TSCA:

- Pesticides
- Foods and food additives
- Drugs
- Cosmetics
- Tobacco and tobacco products
- Nuclear materials
- Munitions

That's a lot of toxic chemicals in our environment![1] And only about 200 of them have actually been tested by the EPA.[2]

In addition to the over 85,500 known chemicals in the environment, there are also high levels of heavy metals, once out of reach deep within the earth, but which now have been mined and unearthed as a result of industrialization. What was once a benign and non-existent threat is now a pervasive threat and one that results in a vicious cycle of re-entry into the environment. These chemicals and heavy metals are found in the soil, pesticides, herbicides, fungicides, and fertilizers; they are in our air and in the food we eat. Those in the soil wash into our lakes, rivers, finding their way into our aquafers and enter our bodies when we drink water. We breathe them in through air fresheners, fumes from cleaning products, and air pollution, and we ingest them through our food, as well as absorb them through our skin in our personal hygiene and skin care products. Once they are in our system, our bodies must metabolize them and excrete them, and then they are back in the environment to start the process all over again.[3]

Herein lies a tremendous problem: we are ingesting more than we are excreting. Many of our diseases are a direct result of these toxic chemicals, substances, and heavy metals in our bodies: inflammation, neurological disorders (Alzheimer's, Parkinson's), digestive disorders, cognitive disorders, autoimmune diseases, cancer, and most other serious health conditions.[4]

Remember, our bodies are beautifully designed to create health, not disease. However, when we eat genetically modified organisms, hormone and antibiotic-laced meats and poultry, pesticide- and herbicide-laden vegetables, use toxic cleaning products, plastic containers that leach chemicals into our food and water, and cosmetics and personal care products filled with chemicals, it is more than our bodies can handle at one time. In other words, we are taking in more toxins than our bodies can process. Thus, these toxins take up residence in our cells, causing significant health issues and damage to our DNA.

In January 2017, the CDC issued its Fourth National Report on Human Exposure to Environmental Chemicals, *Updated Tables, January 2017, Volume One, Volume Two*, identifying and providing details on 308 chemicals found in blood serum and urine samples in the U.S. population.[5] That's 308 chemicals and heavy metals found in our bodies that do not belong there and that our bodies must work hard to expel; if not expelled, these substances cause serious health issues.

As regards heavy metals such as mercury, lead, arsenic, and cadmium, they often mimic the "good" trace minerals in our body, competing with them, making them ineffective and interfering with necessary cellular functions in the body. These weaken the body's immune function, contribute to weight loss resistance, cause oxidative stress, and damage the DNA. They have been shown to cause cancer as well as having been identified as co-carcinogens causing mutations and disruptions to cellular processes.[6]

Another problem as it relates to environmental toxins, and heavy metals in particular, is that it could be transgenerational. "The concept known as transgenerational epigenetics, and which has been proven in numerous studies, says that an exposure to a toxin can cause an illness to future generations even if the individual is never exposed to the toxin again."[7] I eluded to this in Chapters 1 and 2 when I discussed how traditional cultures that did not partake of western industrialized foods required a period of extra nutrition prior to marriage for both the women and the men. I also mentioned a study that found that metabolic changes as a result of processed foods could be passed down. I now want to further explain how this process works in our DNA.

A very important and critical metabolic process our bodies perform each day is called methylation. This process happens more than a billion times per second in every cell and in every organ of the body. Put simply, life would not exist without this process. It is an extremely complex process, but in its simplest term, it is when a molecule passes a methyl group, which consists of one carbon atom linked to three hydrogen atoms, to another molecule. It is a fairly basic process, but one that is absolutely critical. These processes create many necessary substances that our bodies need each day such as creatinine, as well as metabolize certain other substances in the body; methylation also influences the production of ATP, which is the energy unit in the cell.[8]

Methylation affects every tissue and every system in the body, but it affects certain systems more than others. These systems are the brain and the production of neurotransmitters. Because methylation affects the body's ability to detoxify, when there is a disruption in the methylation process it contributes to neurological disorders such as autism spectrum disorders, attention deficit and hyperactive disorder, Alzheimer's, and Parkinson's, and other cognitive and behavioral disorders.[9]

So what does this have to do with "transgenerational" and what does that term mean exactly? Because methylation works at the level of DNA, it is a vital process during fetal development, turning on or turning off the expression of a gene. However, when heavy metals are present, they attach to the methyl bonds and can interfere with the cellular function or these heavy metals can block the cellular function altogether. This type of process is referred to as epigenetics and is a new and emerging field of study wherein we are learning our environment can turn on or turn off the expression of a gene. In other words, when these natural processes are disrupted because of toxin exposure, they can turn on genes that produce a particular disease that were once turned off. Our toxic environment – food, water, air, products – can turn on the expression of a gene to produce cancer, for instance, that would not have been turned on in the absence of these toxins.[10]

What this means is that the chance of contracting a disease is influenced by defects in methylation caused by toxins and you can pass these now defective genes onto your children and they can pass it on to their children. What you eat now, what you breathe in now, what you slather on your skin now, can affect your grandchildren because of the changes within the DNA caused by these toxins. Mike Adams said it best:

> A full understanding of this phenomenon should cause immediate alarm in the mind of anyone reading this. Epigenetic inheritance of toxic side effects from dietary exposure to heavy metals means that *toxicity is trans-generational.* This means that the toxic environment in which we live today will negatively impact future generations for an unknown number of generations *even if we eliminate all exposure starting tomorrow*[11] (emphasis his).

Let that sink in for a moment.

There is already a path in place that has set up the great-grandchildren of today's young adult to be faced with severe neurological and mental disorders, infertility, and other disastrous conditions which will require an abundance of medical care for their life.[12] This information is particularly important for those of child-bearing age. Detoxifying and restoring their bodies to real health through real food prior to conception is more important than ever.

I do want to offer one caveat here; if you suspect that you have heavy metal toxicity, such as mercury or lead, the process of detoxification can be difficult and toxic. A diet and lifestyle as free of these toxins as possible will allow your body to naturally detoxify over time; however, for those with significant health issues due to heavy metal toxicity, do not attempt to detoxify without the assistance of a naturopathic doctor or other medical doctor well-versed in heavy metal detoxification or what is called chelation therapy. Seek the help of an experienced medical professional if you need to detoxify from heavy metal toxicity.

Each time a man stands up for an ideal, or acts to improve the lot of others, or strikes out against injustice, he sends forth a tiny ripple of hope, and crossing each other from a million different centers of energy and daring, those ripples build a current that can sweep down the mightiest walls of oppression and resistance.
Robert F. Kennedy

As we come to the bottom of the rabbit hole, I know the red pill has been hard to swallow. What I have outlined here are only the highlights of deep and complex subjects. Yet, I trust that you have come to see how ignorant bliss and looking the other way have deleterious effects on our health; it also makes us culpable. Those in control of our food supply and our medical system are more concerned with profits than they are with the health of you or your children. It is up to you to take charge of your health.

Clarion Call

As a society, we are at a crossroads. As Christians, we are behind the eight-ball. While you may not want to become an activist who tries to influence policy, you *can* make different choices for you and for your family that will impact the health of future generations. It's not too late.

In this culture rife with the pervasive attitude of refusal to accept responsibility for one's actions, it is more important than ever that we reverse that trend. It is more important than ever that we do what is right for our families, our future generations, our environment, and our animals.

As Christians, we especially should adhere to a diet and life-style that is free of adulterated, toxic food, air, and water. Our choices matter to God. Perhaps you were unaware of the realities of industrialized food; now you know truth and you can't unknow it. You now have a responsibility and moral obligation to protect your children and your grandchildren and protect the lives of the animals God has placed in our care. We will be held accountable one day. It is time to accept responsibility for our health and for the health of our children. It is time to turn from dong what is right in our own mind and looking to the One Who created it all and examine our choices in light of His imperatives.

We are not without hope.

Part II
Hope and Healing

Hope is the thing with feathers that perches in the soul – and sings the tunes without the words – and never stops at all.
Emily Dickinson

7 | The Hope-Filled Journey

Hope deferred makes the heart sick,
But desire fulfilled is a tree of life.
Proverbs 13:12

Take a deep breath.

We have covered a lot of unsavory truths thus far. It is time to emerge from the rabbit hole, step into the light, and realize that there is hope.

I, once again, want to take you into my classroom for another, very short lesson in poetry. Everything about a poem contributes to the meaning and purpose of the poet, including structure. Mueller, at the age of 15, fled World War II Europe with her family; she knows a little something about hope. Enjoy this delightful gem.

Hope
By Lisel Mueller

It hovers in dark corners
before the lights are turned on,
　it shakes sleep from its eyes
　and drops from mushroom gills,
　　it explodes in the starry heads
　　of dandelions turned sages,
　　　it sticks to the wings of green angels
　　　that sail from the tops of maples.

It sprouts in each occluded eye
of the many-eyed potato,
  it lives in each earthworm segment
  surviving cruelty,
    it is the motion that runs
    from the eyes to the tail of a dog.
      it is the mouth that inflates the lungs
      of the child that has just been born.

It is the singular gift
We cannot destroy in ourselves,
The argument that refutes death,
The genius that invents the future,
All we know of God.

It is the serum which makes us swear
Not to betray one another;
It is in this poem, trying to speak.

Why do we so often take hope for granted? We hope our team wins. We hope we get that promotion. We hope it doesn't rain on our outdoor party. We hope. We hope. We hope in many trivial things; but we take for granted that there are signs of real hope all around us. The eye of the potato is the life inside waiting to burst forth; it is in the seeds of the dandelion and the maple tree waiting for the warmth of the earth to release the life they contain. It is in the excitement of your furry friend and in the first breath of a newborn.

Hope. We all need it. We need real hope that promises life and health and healing. Without it, we wither and die. With it, we thrive, like a tree planted by streams of water. It is, indeed, a gift. It is yours for the taking. The structure in the first two stanzas suggests infinity and so it is with hope, real hope. There is an infinite supply.

8

Wellness:
An Act of Worship

There are no unsacred places;
there are only sacred places and desecrated places.
Wendell Berry

Whether, then, you eat or drink or whatever you do,
do all to the glory of God.
1 Corinthians 10:31

When I think back to the garden, when man fell from grace, and sin and disease entered the world, I am in awe at God's mercy upon us. For in that moment, when all seemed lost, He had made provision for our nourishment and for our health. In fact, He put this plan in place before the fall, at the very beginning of creation, *Then God said, 'Let the earth sprout vegetation: plants yielding seed, and fruit trees on the earth bearing fruit after their kind with seed in them;' and it was so. The earth brought forth vegetation, plants yielding seed after their kind, and trees bearing fruit with seed in them, after their kind; and God saw that it was good* (Gen. 1:11-12). It was good!

In these verses, we find the charge of "plants yielding seeds after their own kind." It is clear that our current food system is very far removed from what God originally intended. It was good and it was for our good. Now, our food is adulterated, contaminated, and crossed with other species; and it is not good. Rather, it is harmful, which is why we need to make sure that our food is free of contaminants and not genetically modified or engineered.

Every plant, vegetable, herb, fruit, grain, nut, seed, and eventually animal products (Genesis 9:3), were pronounced good by our Creator. They were perfect just as He created them, bursting with diversity and nutrients necessary and essential for life; theirs and ours. Vibrant life! Abundant life! Can you imagine with me the beauty of it all? Can you feel the nourishment it provides? Does a spirit of worship well up within you? It does me!

In Judaism, mealtime is a time of great importance. Food is considered a gift from God and with the blessing of the food, before and after consumption, the physical act of eating becomes a spiritual event as one acknowledges where their sustenance comes from. The family table is a central focus in Judaism; it is the place where tradition is taught and nurtured and allowed to perpetuate. The family table and the experience of eating together is of such significance in Jewish tradition that the table is compared to the altar in the ancient Holy Temple in Jerusalem.

As Christians, the Holy Spirit resides within us and our bodies are not our own; we belong to Him (1 Corinthians 6:19-20). As the bride of Christ, we are betrothed to Him. I think sometimes we forget that. Think of your relationship with your spouse. Do you want to please him or her? Of course, you do. When you love another person, the things you do and the decisions you make naturally flow out of that love. The same holds true with our love for Christ. We are His and in His grace and mercy and goodness and kindness He has given us the ingredients we need to keep our bodies healthy and He has designed our bodies to lean toward health. He desires that for you.

We are created in His image. It is easy to get caught up in life and reach for any product that is fast and simple to prepare. However, we must ask the question: is this nourishing for my body? Will it impart life to my body, or will it erode the life within my body? Taking care of our bodies is an act of worship and a demonstration of love for our Creator who designed our bodies with the beautifully innate ability to heal itself given the right ingredients!

Preparing meals for your family is an act of worship. It is possible to imbue this task and the food with love. Do you remember meals at your grandmother's house? Meals at my grandmother's house were always memorable: one, because extended family was gathered around and it was always a good time; and two, because the food was just so good! I believe that is directly related to the fact that she poured her nurturing spirit into the food; the overwhelming love she had for her family was infused into the food she prepared, which we consumed and we were nourished, not just by the meal, but with the love with which it was prepared.

It is possible to use this time of food preparation for meditation and reflection and prayer; that energy will flow into the food that you serve your family or your guests. When we make a point of using that time to pray and meditate on scripture, the act of preparing food is no longer a mundane activity, but a spiritual one. By focusing on the purpose of those actions, you will begin to see the beauty in the bounty we have been given. When you begin to integrate prayer and scripture with the physical act of food preparation, you will transfer that love into the task of nurturing your family.

9

Real Food is
Real Good

Let food be thy medicine and let thy medicine be food.
Hippocrates

*God in His infinite wisdom, neglected nothing and
if we would eat our food without trying to improve,
change, or refine it, thereby destroying its life-giving
elements, it would meet all requirements of the body.*
Jethro Kloss

We spent a good portion of Part 1 discussing what not to eat; now let's explore what nutrient dense food looks like. Processed, food-like products are not real food. Real food *is* the ingredient. However, quality matters, too. Once your taste buds acclimate to real food, there's no going back because that other stuff will taste like cardboard.

I was at a seaside restaurant having lunch with a dear friend, dining on fresh caught tuna and fresh produce and fresh fruit from a local farmer, savoring every morsel when I look up and my friend is sitting with arms crossed, staring at me with a grin from ear to ear.

What?
I'm just enjoying watching you enjoy your meal.
Blush.
Is it that noticeable?
Yes, it is!

Oh! This is so good! As I continue to relish every bite.

I don't know why this memory is so affixed in my mind, except that I do remember the food being incredibly good and apparently it showed and well, I do so enjoy good food!

Yes, real food is really, really good! And it doesn't have to be complicated; however, quality does matter because we need our food to be as nutrient dense as possible.

Nutrient Dense Foods

Our bodies were designed to desire foods in their whole, natural state. Our bodies are beautifully and intricately created to function optimally based on specific nutritional requirements. From the beginning of time, the biological and physiological needs of the body have been foods that are nutrient dense. Prior to the Industrial Revolution, we did not partake of any industrialized foods, and the diet was primarily free of sugars. Foods were fresh and local, unprocessed, unrefined, and free of hormones and antibiotics and chemicals. Food was what is now referred to as "clean." (It is a sad commentary on our society that we have to qualify food as either clean or contaminated.) The soil was rich and fertile, teaming with minerals which are taken up by the plants the people and the animals ate.

Our ancestors, epitomized by the indigenous peoples Dr. Price studied, had a diet of varied fruits and vegetables, some animal food; depending on their location, it included land mammals, seafood, eggs, raw dairy and fermented dairy products. It was a combination of cooked and uncooked foods. They used all parts of the animal, including bones for making broth, and organs meats, which were preferred. Fat from these animals was also a part of their diet.[1]

Dr. Price discovered that because of rich soil fertility the foods these people groups consumed contained "at least four times the minerals and water-soluble vitamins, and TEN times the fat-soluble vitamins found in animal fats (vitamin A, vitamin D, and Activator X, now thought to be vitamin K_2) as the average American diet."[2] This ratio is undoubtedly much greater today.

This is why, long before the discovery of vitamins and minerals, these peoples lived without vitamin deficiencies.

The diet of traditional cultures contained anywhere from 30 to 80 percent of the daily intake of calories from fat; however, only about 4 percent of those fat calories came from polyunsaturated fats which are naturally occurring in grains, legumes, nuts, fish, animal fats, and vegetables. The majority of the fat calories they consumed were saturated or monounsaturated. And the ratio of omega-3 to omega-6 essential fatty acids was about equal. Today, there is a big disparity in that ratio, with omega-6 making up the bulk of fatty acids.[3]

It is important, also, to remember that ancient cultures and those that Dr. Price studied were diligent and methodical in providing special nutrient-dense periods of feeding, including animal foods, for young couples prior to marriage, both young men and young women. As well, children received special attention when it came to dietary needs. This knowledge was passed down from generation to generation.[4]

All of the chronic diseases that we suffer from today are a result of industrialized, adulterated, contaminated food and the ever increasing use of pharmaceuticals: autoimmune conditions, diabetes, heart disease, cancer, digestive disorders, neurological disorders, dementia are all modern diseases. With a rare exception, they did not exist, especially on a chronic basis, until 100 years ago. That is thousands of years that humanity was not plagued by chronic conditions.

Protein

Proteins are the building blocks of our bodies. The word protein derives from the Greek word *proteus* meaning primary importance.[5] While the body requires 22 amino acids, the body assembles and utilizes about 50,000 different proteins which are necessary to form muscles, organs, flesh, and nerves. Enzymes and antibodies are specialized proteins.[6]

The body has the ability to make all of the 22 amino acids except for eight "essential" amino acids which are found in food. When these eight amino acids are present in the food, the body can manufacture the remaining 14 amino acids; but when just one of the eight is missing or low, the body cannot synthesize the other proteins even when protein intake is high. All eight of the essential proteins must be ingested in order for the body to use any of them. It's all or nothing.

Animal meat is a complete protein, meaning that it provides all eight of the essential amino acids. When we do not get the protein we need, we begin to loose heart muscle. However, without the presence of fat, the protein cannot be properly utilized, thus the reason protein and fat are usually found together in milk, meat, eggs, and fish. Proteins found in vegetables are not complete proteins, meaning they do not contain all eight essential amino acids. Properly prepared (soaked, sprouted, or fermented) grains, nuts, seeds, and legumes are good sources of protein in the vegetable kingdom. A combination of these along with a small amount of animal protein is important.

Vegetarians, or those following a plant-based diet, will argue that meat is bad for you; however, this is a dangerous stance. According to Sally Fallon Morell, a nutritional researcher:

> Not only is it difficult to obtain adequate protein on a diet devoid of animal products, but such a diet often leads to deficiencies in many important minerals as well. This is because a largely vegetarian diet lacks fat-soluble catalysts needed for mineral absorption. Furthermore, phytates in grains block absorption of calcium, iron, zinc, copper, and magnesium. Unless grains are properly prepared to neutralize phytates, the body may be unable to assimilate these minerals. We should not underestimate the damages of deficiencies in these minerals.[7]

Phosphorus, zinc, and iron are other important minerals only present in meat. Many chronic conditions can be linked to deficiencies in vitamins and minerals.

Additionally, the form of B_{12} which is bioavailable to the body is only found in animal products. The body stores B_{12} in the body for two to five years; after that, deficiencies begin to result and these deficiencies have been linked to pernicious anemia, neurological disorders, mental and psychological disorders. Supplementation often is not effective because specialized proteins present in the stomach do not recognize the B_{12} in supplements.[8]

Protein powders are made from protein isolates of soy, casein, whey, and egg whites. This is a highly processed "food" from ingredients that are likely genetically engineered or from factory farmed animals. The process denatures the amino acids and renders them essentially useless, at the same time creating MSG, which is a neurotoxin and because it is not an "added" ingredient it is not required to be labeled. In addition, "soy protein isolates are high in mineral-blocking phytates, thyroid-depressing phytoestrogens, and potent enzyme inhibitors that depress growth and cause cancer."[9] In short, protein powders are not real food, not bioavailable to the body, and a waste of money.

Animal products are necessary; they are building blocks for the body and certain amino acids are necessary for brain development and neurological functions. The body cannot function properly without animal protein. It is important to remember that protein should be eaten along with animal fats which supply the vitamins A and D that are needed for the assimilation of the protein in the body. Using meat bones to make broth is another way of getting these proteins into your diet and is especially helpful if you are on a tight budget.

I hope that I have already convinced you not to eat conventional meat, poultry, and eggs from factory farms. Not only are they contaminated, but their nutritional value is inferior, at best, to that of pastured animals. It is well worth the effort to find local sources for meats, poultry, and eggs which are raised humanely on pasture.

When sourcing fish, avoid all farmed fish, they have been fed antibiotics and inappropriate feed such as soy and corn meal. Cold water fish, deep sea fish, are especially good choices as they are rich in omega-3 fat soluble vitamins; wild caught is best. Again, avoid farm raised fish of all types. Also, avoid scavenger fish such as carp and catfish as they are extremely contaminated.

When cooking meats, avoid high temperature cooking as these may contain carcinogens. The best options are raw, rare, or braised in water or stock. Avoid processed meats such as sausage and luncheon meats that are filled with preservatives and bacon that contains nitrates.

Fats

Fats, particularly saturated fats, have been vilified for 50 years, but the indoctrination started 100 years ago when Proctor and Gamble realized that their cotton industry produced a lot of waste product, so let's just turn this sludge into cooking fat to replace traditional animal fats. (I described this process in Chapter 2). Initially P&G used this product in candles, but with the advent of electricity, they needed a new market for this waste, so along came Crisco and a massive and creative marketing campaign which included a cookbook using this new "fat."[10] Who thinks of using cotton (waste) for food?! Granted, animals can graze on cotton plants after harvest, but people? Botanically, it is in the vegetable genus, but it is not food for human consumption.

In the 1950s, Ancel Keys postulated that saturated fats and cholesterol in the diet caused heart disease. While there were many flaws in his research and data that highlighted these flaws in subsequent research, the Proctor and Gambles of the vegetable oil industry who would benefit from Keys' flawed research used this as an opportunity to push the vegetable oil and other fat substitutes like margarine.[11] The many studies over these past 50 plus years which demonstrate that animal and vegetable fats do not cause heart disease have been demonized and their findings quietly subverted, until recently.

Saturated fats from pastured animal and organic vegetable sources are good for you! They are a concentrated source of energy, an important constituent in cell membranes, and they play a role in regulating hormones. When consumed as part of a meal, (remember fats should be eaten with protein) they slow nutrient absorption which turns off the hunger trigger and satiates the body for longer. Fat-soluble vitamins, like A, D, E, and K, require fat to make these vitamins bioavailable to the body. They are required for mineral absorption and many other biological processes.[12]

There are three primary classifications of fats: saturated, monounsaturated, and polyunsaturated.

- Saturated fats are very stable and generally do not go rancid when subjected to high heat in cooking. They are mostly solid at room temperature. They are found primarily in animal fats and tropical oils.

- Monounsaturated fats are also fairly stable and can be subjected to low amounts of heat without becoming rancid. They are liquid at room temperature. They are found in olive oil as well as oil from almonds, pecans, cashews, peanuts, and avocados.

- Polyunsaturated fats, omega-3 and omega-6 are "essential" fatty acids and cannot be produced by the body and we must get them from food. They can go rancid very easily and should never be heated. They remain liquid even when refrigerated.

All animal and vegetable fats contain a combination of these fatty acids in varying ratios with animal fats containing 40-60% saturated fats.[13]

At the turn of the 20th century, heart disease was extremely rare and the majority of fats in the diet came from animal fats such as butter, tallow, lard, and coconut oil which contain mainly saturated and monounsaturated fats. However, our modern diet contains primarily polyunsaturated fats (industry vegetable oils produced at high temperatures – see Chapter 2). The intake of polyunsaturated fat should be no more than 4% of caloric total with a ratio of 1.5% omega-3 to 2.5% omega-6 intake. Yet, in our modern diet the total polyunsaturated intake is approximately 30% of calories.[14]

Polyunsaturated fats are fragile and should never be exposed to high heat because this causes the fats to oxidize and become rancid, which creates free radicals which then cause damage to the DNA and RNA which leads to a host of problems within the body such as premature aging, autoimmune diseases, Parkinson's disease, Lou Gehrig's disease and Alzheimer's. To add insult to injury, most commercial vegetable oils are high in omega-6 which can result in problems with blood clotting, inflammation, high blood pressure, immune dysfunction, digestive issues, cancer, sexual reproduction, and weight gain.[15]

The ratio of omega-3 to omega-6 in commercial products has practically eliminated omega-3s and dramatically increased the amount of omega-6s, "....organic eggs from hens allowed to feed on insects and green plants can contain omega-6 and omega-3 fatty acids in the beneficial ration of approximately one-to-one, but commercial supermarket eggs from hens fed grains can contain as much as nineteen times more omega-6 than omega-3!"[16] I cannot stress enough the importance of consuming animal products that are raised on pasture, in their natural environment, and free of hormones and antibiotics!

Saturated fats are important to the physiological processes in the body and they are particularly important for heart and brain health. Per Morell:[17]

- Saturated fatty acids constitute at least 50% of the cell membranes, giving them necessary stiffness and integrity.

- They play a vital role in bone health. For calcium to be effectively incorporated into the skeletal structure, at least 50% of the dietary fats should be saturated.

- They lower Lp(a), a substance in the blood that indicates proneness to heart disease.

- They enhance the immune system.

- They are needed for the proper utilization of essential fatty acids. Omega-3 fatty acids are better retained in the tissues when the diet is rich in saturated fats.

- The fat around the heart is highly saturated and acts as a reserve in times of stress; thus the need for saturated fats for heart health.

- They have important antimicrobial properties which protect us against harmful microorganisms in the digestive tract.

Saturated fats are not the enemy; rather, they are your friend. Saturated fats are not the cause of our modern disease; rather they play a vital role in promoting and maintaining an optimally functioning body, the way it was designed. Modern industrialization has vilified the nutrient dense foods of thousands of years and in the last 100 years has replaced them with industrial waste and dangerous ratios of fat intake our Creator never intended for us to consume.

The only substance more demonized than saturated fats is cholesterol. What is cholesterol and what is its purpose? It is a natural healing substance produced by the body which has many functions. According to Morell:[18]

- Along with saturated fats, cholesterol provides necessary stiffness and stability for cell membranes.

- Cholesterol acts a precursor to corticosteroids, hormones that help us deal with stress and protect the body against heart disease and cancer, and to the sex hormones testosterone, estrogen, and progesterone.

- Cholesterol is a precursor to vitamin D.

- Necessary bile salts are made from cholesterol.

- It acts as an antioxidant.

- Cholesterol is needed for proper function of serotonin.

- Mother's milk is especially rich in cholesterol and contains a special enzyme that helps the baby utilize this nutrient. Babies and children need cholesterol-rich foods through their growing years to ensure proper development of the brain and nervous system.

- Cholesterol plays a role in maintaining the health of the intestinal wall. Low cholesterol (vegetarian) diets can lead to leaky gut and other intestinal disorders.

The consumption of free radicals created by the improper processing of polyunsaturated fats, excessive consumption of vegetable oils, hydrogenated fats, sugar, white flour, mineral and vitamin deficiencies, the elimination of antimicrobial fats from the diet which prevent the pathogenic bacteria and viruses that cause arterial plaque requires that cholesterol rush in to save the day, only to be lowered by satin drugs (which are only effective for 1% of the people and they have over 300 side effects.[19]) and low cholesterol diets. It is utter insanity. Heart disease will not be prevented without the reversal of these trends and the consumption of saturated fats and cholesterol from grass-fed, pastured meat, poultry, and eggs and diets rich in vitamins and minerals and by eliminating processed foods and high intake of carbohydrates.[20]

Avoid all low-fat foods; they are one of the worst substances for your health. The fat has been removed, along with the wonderful flavor, and replaced with sugar, to add flavor. Avoid all hydrogenated oils as well; the production process converts these into *trans-fats*. It is the sugar, these rancid oils, and refined car-bohydrates that are the scourge of our modern society.

Carbohydrates

Carbohydrates are the *starches* and *sugars* produced by all plants where proteins and fats synthesize them into usable constituents. There are many forms of sugar. Table sugar is the simple sugar, sucrose, and any additive ending in *–ose* is a sugar. Sucrose is a disaccharide which breaks down during digestion into glucose and fructose. Glucose is the sugar in the blood. Fructose is primarily found in fruits and high fructose corn syrup.[21]

Complex sugars are found in beans and legumes and they are difficult to digest without first properly preparing them by soaking (see the section of proper preparation of grains below) because we do not possess the enzymes necessary to break these complex sugars into simple sugars, or disaccharides.[22]

Conversely, humans are able to digest starches that are poly-saccharides which are exclusively glucose, a necessary substance for many different processes in the body. It would seem that we need sugar since glucose is necessary for energy production, and for motion; however, the body is capable of producing glucose without ingesting large quantities of sugar or starches.[23]

As with the elimination of fats in the diet in the last 100 years, we have also seen a rise in the amount of refined carbo-hydrates and a rise in the consumption of sugar. The process of refining carbohydrates strips them of the necessary vitamins, minerals, fiber, protein, and enzymes and it concentrates the starches without the buffer these vital nutrients provide and which are necessary for proper digestion. Without these nutri-ents, the body must reach into its own stores of the necessary constituents, further depleting the body. Refined carbohydrates have been referred to as "empty" calories, but for the reasons stated, the more appropriate term given them by Sally Fallon Morell is "negative" calories due to the draining effect on the body.[24] This sets the stage for the metabolic changes I have discussed earlier that gets passed down to future generations.

> The all-important level of glucose in the blood is regulated by a finely tuned mechanism involving the insulin secretions from the pancreas and hormones from several glands, including the adrenal glands and the thyroid. When sugars and starches are eaten in their natural, unrefined form, as part of a meal containing nourishing fats and protein, they are digested slowly and enter the bloodstream at a moderate rate over a period of several hours. . . . When properly working, this marvelous blood sugar regulation process provides our cells with a steady, even supply of glucose. The body is kept on an even keel, so to speak, both physically and emotionally.
>
> But when we consume *refined* sugars and starches, particularly alone, without fats or proteins, they enter the blood stream in a rush, causing a sudden increase in blood sugar. The body's regulation mechanism kicks into high gear, flooding the bloodstream with insulin and other hormones to bring blood sugar levels down to acceptable levels. Repeated onslaughts of sugar will eventually disrupt this finely tuned process, causing some elements to remain in a constant state of activity and others to become worn out and inadequate to do the job. The situation is exacerbated by the fact that a diet high in refined carbohydrates will also be deficient in vitamins, minerals and enzymes, those bodybuilding elements that keep the glands and organs in good repair. When the endocrine system becomes disturbed, numerous other pathological conditions soon manifest – degenerative disease, allergies, obesity, alcoholism, drug addition, depression, learning disabilities, and behavioral problems.[25]

This yo-yo effect will result in either a person becoming diabetic (chronic too high blood sugar) or hypoglycemic (chronic too low blood sugar). Same cause. Different affects. Both have deleterious effects on long-term health.

Our bodies were designed to need "whole" foods that are in their original, unrefined, natural state. Properly prepared whole grains are rich in vitamin E and B vitamins and minerals our bodies need to function properly. As discussed in Chapter 2, refining of whole grains strips them of these nutrients that are then "replaced" with synthetic versions that our bodies do not recognize and are therefore, useless. Additionally, not all of the B vitamins that are removed are added back in disrupting the processes dependent on all of the B vitamins together in concert.

Prior to the 20th century, sugar was moderately consumed and it was always a natural sweetener such as sugar or paste made from dates, raw honey, or maple syrup, all of which are packed with many vitamins and minerals. The consumption of sugar in the last 100 years has skyrocketed. So how much sugar are we consuming?

> According to the United States Department of Agriculture, the average American consumes about 150 to 170 pounds of refined sugars each year! That means most of us consume our whole body weight or more in sugar. Another way of thinking of it is that we're single handedly downing 30-34 five-pound bags of refined sugar each, adding up to almost ½ pound per day. Eat a full teaspoon of sugar every 24 minutes every day of your life and now you have an idea of the average sugar intake.
>
> And if that's not startling enough, remember that the average includes all of those folks who are health conscious and watch their sugar intake. So for every person that eats only 5 pounds of a sugar a year, someone else is eating a mind-boggling 295 pounds. To put that in perspective, in the early 1900s ...we only ate 4 pounds of sugar per year on average.[26]

This comes in many forms: sugary drinks/sodas, fruit juice, cereals and refined carbohydrates. Two out of three adults and one out of three children in the United States are overweight or obese. In the last 30 years, adolescent obesity rates have tripled and childhood obesity rates have doubled. It is estimated that the obesity rate for all 50 states will be 44% by 2030. The consumption of refined carbohydrates and the diseases associated with the consumption of refined carbohydrates is reaching epidemic proportions.

Dairy

There is a much controversy surrounding the consumption of milk these days; it is quite the hot topic. However, I posit that the debate surrounds conventional dairy and not raw dairy as our Creator designed it to be consumed. The dairy found in your local grocery is from cows in CAFOs (Chapter 4) and should be completely avoided. These cows have been bred to produce three to four times as much milk as cows raised on pasture, are injected with growth hormones, antibiotics, and plagued with sickness.

Raw milk contains: lactic-acid producing bacteria which protect against pathogens; enzymes which assist the body to assimilate all of the minerals in dairy – calcium, magnesium, phosphorus, potassium, sodium, and sulfur; B vitamins, vitamins D, A, and K; proteins and saturated fats. Raw milk from pastured cows is healthy food.

Conventional dairy is pasteurized, effectively destroying all of the protective bacteria, enzymes, vitamins, and minerals, as well as denaturing the proteins and fats. This practice began with the flawed science of Louis Pasteur (Chapter 5) and while his science was flawed and debunked, the practice continues. The many outbreaks of salmonella[27] in the last several decades have all occurred in pasteurized milk.

The process of fermentation, found in all traditional cultures, partially breaks down the lactose in dairy and predigests the protein casein. The products of this process, such as kefir, yogurt, sour cream, buttermilk, cultured butter, and raw cheeses, are generally well-tolerated by those who have issues with fresh milk. For those with severe lactose intolerance, ghee, or clarified butter, is a good option. Raw cheeses contain all of the enzymatic activity of raw dairy; conventional cheeses, however, are made from pasteurized milk, with emulsifiers, phosphates, and hydrogenated oils and should be strictly avoided. Also, unheated cheese is more digestible than heated.

Goat's milk can be an excellent alternative to cow's milk; it is less allergenic, more easily digestible, and has many of the same nutrients as cow's milk and it can be fermented in the same way as cow's milk to make yogurt, kefir, and cheese, for instance.

States have varying laws concerning the purchase of raw dairy, but it is well worth the effort to source this; if you cannot source raw dairy, it is best to avoid conventional dairy and products made from conventional dairy altogether. See the Resources section for information on how to find raw dairy in your area.

The Three Amigos:
Enzymes, Vitamins, and Minerals

Modern science has discovered what traditional cultures have always intuitively known. The food we eat contains life-giving properties. The vast array of vitamins, minerals, and enzymes in the food we eat and the intricate processes they perform can never be replicated in pill form. These three amigos play very well together and, in fact, depend on each other for the ability to carry out their designated duties. Enzymes are proteins that are involved in almost all biochemical processes in the body and this activity depends on vitamins and minerals.

There are three types of enzymes: digestive, metabolic, and food. Digestive enzymes are primarily produced in the pancreas and they assist the body in breaking down food into digestible particles. The metabolic enzymes are involved in all bodily processes from breathing to supporting the immune system to assisting the body in eliminating toxins. Food enzymes are those found in certain raw foods and in fermented foods and aid in digestion.

Many disease processes can be traced to vitamin and mineral deficiencies and can, therefore, be reversed or halted by adopting a diet that is rich in nutrient dense foods replete with vitamins, minerals, and enzymes. However, in order for food to be nutrient dense, the quality of the soil and the farming practices used, are crucial. Our modern industrialized food system has stripped the soil of nutrients, genetic engineering has destroyed the seed, and processing with high heat methods, all leave the food we consume devoid of any real nutrition, devoid of the vitamins, minerals, and enzymes necessary for life.

We are so programmed to take a pill or drink a chemical cocktail liquid pill and call it a "protein shake" or "meal replacement." A pill will not fix what ails you. Food is medicine, and if nutrient dense, it has all of the compliments of vitamins and minerals and proteins and fats and enzymes that our bodies need. Our bodies are not designed to recognize and assimilate synthetic "vitamins." Supplementation should not be the first go to remedy; rather correcting what you eat should be your first go to remedy. And supplements are expensive; use the money you would normally spend on supplements and invest in quality food.

The American Journal of Clinical Nutrition, in a published paper "Food Synergy: An Operational Concept for Understanding Nutrition" emphasizes the importance of obtaining nutrition from whole foods: "A person or animal eating a diet consisting solely of purified nutrients in their Dietary Reference Intake amounts, without the benefit of the coordination inherent in food, may not thrive and probably will not have optimal health. This review argues for the primacy of food over supplements in meeting nutritional requirements of the population."[28]

The authors of the study further stated, "The concept of food synergy is based on the proposition that the interrelations between constituents in foods are significant. This significance is dependent on the balance between constituents within the food, how well the constituents survive digestion, and the extent to which they appear biologically active at the cellular level."[29]

Synthetic, isolated forms of nutrients usually do not have the same effect on the body as they do when in their whole state and present with other constituents in the food. Often industrial processing forms a different compound entirely. Folic acid, for instance, the compound found in vitamins, is not the same as the naturally occurring folate and the human body does a very poor job of converting folic acid into folate. Additionally, most studies conclude that supplementing with multivitamins is a bad idea in that they either provide no benefit or they may cause harm. Part of the problem is that they contain too much of nutrients that can be toxic such as folic acid, calcium, iron, and vitamin E, and not enough of the beneficial nutrients like vitamins D and K_2, and magnesium.[30]

Most Americas are deficient in vitamins A, D, K_2, C and these can be difficult to get from food. However, if you are consuming quality animal fats and fermented vegetables, you should be able to obtain all of these vitamins. As well, most people are deficient in magnesium, and a high quality supplement can prove beneficial.

Lacto-Fermentation

The diets of traditional cultures contained lacto-fermented vegetables, dairy, fruits, and beverages which resulted in foods rich with enzymes and beneficial bacteria. The fermentation process uses beneficial microorganisms which produce enzymes to pre-digest nutritional compounds that would otherwise pass through the digestive tract without being absorbed and increases vitamin levels, including vitamin K. These foods are nutritional powerhouses. Examples include sauerkraut and other vegetable combinations, and fruits, the choices are endless; dairy products such as yogurt, kefir, raw cheese, cultured crème or *cremé fraish*, all of which contain many different strains of probiotics that you can't get from a pill. Someone who is lactose intolerant can safely consume fermented dairy products because the microorganisms feed on the lactose and leave behind galactose, a monosaccharide which can be easily digested. Modern vinegar-based commercial techniques do not produce these same results and these are pasteurized which kills all of the beneficial bacteria. It is a process you can easily do at home. (See Resources)

It bears reiterating here that the fermented dairy products are made from raw dairy. Modern pasteurization methods denature the milk, removing all of the enzymes and beneficial bacteria. Pasteurized milk comes from factory animals which are sick and unhealthy to begin with and the process of heating the milk also alters the protein structure making them unavailable for assimilation by the body. Modern pasteurized dairy should be strictly avoided.

Traditional Preparation of Grains, Nuts, Seeds

Let's face it. We all love grains. Who doesn't love bread? Slathered in butter? Or even better, garlic butter? Or pasta? Or rice? Or oatmeal? We all do, yet, they are slowly killing us.

Modern wheat is a freak of nature. It has been hybridized to the point that the gluten content is exponentially higher than that of ancient wheat such as einkorn, spelt, and teff. If that were not enough, it has been modified by chemical mutagenesis to resist being sprayed with Roundup, which doesn't wash off (Chapter 3). Not only that, it is highly processed using crude means. In short, it is poison.

However, grains, particularly ancient grains, are not inherently bad for you. Nutritionally, whole grains contain proteins, dietary fiber, B vitamins, magnesium, selenium, and iron. Yet, in order for our bodies to access these nutrients, the grains need proper preparation either by sprouting, soaking, or fermenting.

Traditional cultures consumed seeds, nuts, and grains which were first soaked, sprouted, or fermented. This is a necessary process because grains, seeds, and most nuts are protected by a layer of phytic acid and polyphenols (tannins), which are enzyme inhibitors. Since grains, nuts, and seeds germinate, this layer of phytic acid protects the vital nutrients within them that promotes germination.

Humans do not possess the enzymes necessary to break down this layer of phytic acid and tannins, therefore, the nutrients within them are not bioavailable. Also, the phytic acid can bind with calcium, magnesium, iron, and zinc and block their absorption. In order to reduce this layer so that the body can access these nutrients and to neutralize the phytic acid and tannins, nuts, seeds, and grains require special preparation before consumption. These traditional cultures instinctively knew to mimic nature. Having abandoned this process in the modern diet could be a contributing factor to mineral deficiencies.

Soaking

To mimic nature's process of germination, nuts and seeds, with a few exceptions, should be soaked in salt water for 7 to 10 hours, drained and dried in a dehydrator until crisp. An acid such as whey, lemon juice, or raw apple cider vinegar also can be added to the soaking water. If you don't have a dehydrator, this could be done on trays outside in the sun during the summer. I highly recommend purchasing a quality dehydrator for use in a real food kitchen; it is well worth the investment and has many different uses. My grandmother did not own a dehydrator, and neither did the traditional cultures. My grandmother used a piece of sheet metal stretched over two saw-horses to dry every type of food imaginable during the hot, dry summer months. Ancient cultures soaked their grains overnight and left them out in the open air to dry.

For grains, omit the salt; instead use an acid such as whey. apple cider vinegar, lemon juice; Soak overnight, or at least 8-12 hours. This process neutralizes the enzyme inhibitors and reduces the cooking time in half. For grains that are ground into flour without being sprouted first, it is best to use yogurt, kefir, or buttermilk for soaking. For example, if you were going to make biscuits with organic spelt flour, soak in an acid for 8-12 hours before continuing with the recipe. (See Resources)

Sprouting

Traditionally, after grains were cut and harvested in the fields, they were loosely tied together and left to stand overnight in the fields before being threshed which began the germinating process. Today, you can perform this same process by purchasing the whole grain, rinsing the grain in water, leaving to sit for 24 hours, and repeat if necessary, until you begin to see the grain sprout. At that point, you will need a grain mill to grind the grain into flour and use immediately or store in the freezer. Since most of us do not own a grain mill, this is not convenient which is why soaking is necessary.

Fermenting

Fermenting as it relates to nuts, seeds, and grains generally refers to the process used to make sourdough bread. Water is added to flour, covered, and left to sit at room temperature for several days. This is referred to as "wild fermentation" and it will capture the "wild" bacteria and yeast in your home, which always varies by region. However, that process can be a bit tricky if you are new to fermenting. Sourdough starter cultures can be purchased which will almost guarantee success. Again, this process of fermenting the flour will neutralize the enzyme inhibitors. (See Resources)

Soaking, sprouting, and fermenting are also used for lentils, beans, and legumes. These properly prepared foods are an excellent source of carbohydrates, unlike the processed and refined grains and cereals we find in our modern diet that raise blood sugar and contribute to obesity and diabetes. Nuts, seeds, and grains, properly prepared should be consumed in moderation. It should also be noted that these traditional cultures did not feast on grains in the same way that we do. Their diets were low in carbohydrate intake and high in fat and moderate protein.

Salt

Traditional cultures also used salt, though not the kind that we find today in the cardboard tub with a spout. Today's modern table salt is devoid of any of the trace minerals found in salts that are not processed. Sea salt contains about 84 different trace minerals that our bodies need. Modern table salt is mined rock salt which is stripped of all of the trace minerals, bleached so as to have a uniform color, then anti-caking agents are added, which are usually a form of aluminum, and often iodine has been added in as well.

Our bodies need salt and the trace minerals present in unrefined salt are what helps to balance the body's processes, such as blood pressure. People who suffer from high blood pressure are often told to decrease their salt intake, but because our bodies need sodium, this only exacerbates the problem. It is not that we need less salt; it is that we need less refined salt. Seasoning with unrefined sea salt is healthy and necessary. Be aware that a true unrefined sea salt is not white and it does clump; that is the test of real unrefined sea salt.

Quality Matters

To get the best quality and the highest nutrient dense foods, buy locally from farmers who use organic and sustainable practices, cattle ranchers who pasture-raise their cattle, and dairy farmers who also pasture-raise their cows. There are many farmers' markets popping up all over the country now. If you want the best quality food, local markets are where you will find it. You can talk with them, ask them about their practices and know for certain that your food is free of harmful chemicals and that your meat comes from healthy, happy animals. For those who argue that it is more expensive, I say so is ill health. It really is a matter of priorities.

If you do not have access to locally produced food, then you will need to be a savvy shopper. The food industry is a master at marketing. The next time you pick up a package of meat, for instance, pay attention to the label. Often labels will be a picturesque farm setting leading you to believe that the animal who gave its life for that end product was raised humanely. However, as I have already covered, this is not the case. Labels can also be rather misleading and it is helpful to understand what the various terms used in labeling mean. Here is a partial list from sustainabletable.org.[31]

Cage-free	This term is most often applied to egg laying hens, not to poultry raised for meat. As the term implies, hens laying eggs labeled as "cage-free" are raised without using cages, but almost always live inside barns or warehouses. This term does not explain if the birds had any access to the outside, whether any outside area was pasture or a bare lot, or if they were raised entirely indoors in overcrowded conditions. Beak cutting is permitted. No independent third party verification.
Free-range	Defined for poultry meat only. In order to use "free roaming" or "free range" on a poultry meat label the producer must demonstrate to the USDA that poultry have access to the outdoors. However, the type of outdoor access provided (such as pasture or dirt lot), the length of time animals are required to have outdoor access, and how this is verified is not legally defined, and therefore varies greatly from facility to facility. There is no guarantee that birds actually go outside. When used to describe laying hens and other animals, the terms "free range" and "free roaming" are not legally defined at all, and there is no requirement to demonstrate that birds and animals have even had access to the outside, let alone any reference to other management practices. No independent third party verification.

Grass-fed	100% of the diet of grass-fed animals consists of freshly grazed pasture during the growing season and stored grasses (hay or grass silage) during the winter months or drought conditions. This term refers only to the diet of cattle, sheep, goats, and bison. It does not indicate if an animal has been given access to pasture, or if it has been raised in a feedlot and/or given antibiotics or hormones. The USDA definition goes on to state that "if for environmental or health of the animal reasons supplementation can be used if the producer logs the type and amount." Hence, feedlot cattle could be fed harvested forage and supplements, antibiotics and synthetic hormones and still bear the USDA grassfed label. The American Grassfed Association (AGA) has an independent third party certification program available to ranchers. The AGA certified program is recognized by FSIS (the USDA Food Safety and Inspection Service) and verifies a 100 percent forage diet, raised on pasture that has a minimum of 75 percent cover, no confinement, no antibiotics and no added hormones. Meat purchasers seeking truly grassfed meat should source AGA certified products.
Organic	All products sold as "organic" must meet the USDA National Organic Program production and handling standards. Certification is mandatory for farmers selling more than $5,000 of organic products per year, and is verified by an accredited certifying agency. In general, organic production limits the use of chemicals, pesticides, hormones, antibiotics and other inputs. However, it does not strictly define production practices related to space per animal or outdoor access requirements – for example, confinement areas are permitted to fatten organic beef cattle.

Pastured/ Pasture Raised	In general, pasturing is a traditional farming technique where animals are raised outdoors in a humane, ecologically sustainable manner and eat foods that nature intended them to eat. Animals are raised on pasture rather than being fattened on a feedlot or in a confined facility. Note this term is not regulated.
Vegetarian Fed	Animals have been fed a diet free of animal products. This does not mean animals were raised outdoors on pasture or were fed a 100 percent grassfed diet. No independent third party verification.

As you can see, labels are very misleading; it's all about marketing. If you cannot source these products locally, there are now many online stores where you can purchase quality meat and poultry products.

To Drink or Not to Drink

Hydration matters. What you're drinking matters. The quality of what you're drinking matters. So, what are you drinking?

A can of soda contains about 10 teaspoons of sugar! Or, the "diet" variety contains aspartame which is a known neurotoxin. Fruit drinks, especially those marketed to children, often contain as much or more sugar than some sodas. Anything that comes in a can, bottle, or pouch and is flavored contains added sugar or high fructose corn syrup from *Bt* genetically modified corn. Fruit juices are equally dangerous because they are a concentration of fructose. In fact, 12 ounces of orange juice contains as much sugar as a can of soda; some juices contain even more than that.[32]

Coffee and tea are a balancing act. Sweetened specialty coffees are more like a dessert. Exercise restraint. Fair trade, organic coffee is a good choice when consumed in moderation. Organic loose teas have many health benefits as long as you don't load up on the sugar.

Water is always a good choice; however, quality is very important. Many bottled waters are contaminated and the plastic bottles, when exposed to heat such as when being shipped in the trailer of a semi across country, leach toxic chemicals into the water. Tap water, depending on your location, can contain fluoride, which is a neurotoxin, and chlorine. There are a plethora of water filters on the market, so research is necessary to find the one that will work for your situation; they are necessary.

The amount of water you drink is also important. The old standby of eight 8-ounce glasses of water has been deemed inappropriate. One size does not fit all. Too much water is detrimental also, as it puts a strain on the kidneys. A better rule of thumb is to drink half your body weight in ounces each day. For a person weighing 100 pounds, that would be 50 ounces; but again, this is only a guide, and not a hard and fast rule. Your particular circumstances should dictate, but staying adequately hydrated is important for all of the biological processes in our bodies. Water should contain minerals and electrolytes and it should be consumed throughout the day. However, drinking a lot of water before, during, and after a meal, is hard on digestion because the water dilutes the stomach acid needed to digest food. Only small amounts of water should be consumed with a meal and no more than 30 minutes before a meal or two hours after a meal should large amounts of fluids be consumed.

Fermented beverages are always a good choice. Traditional peoples have been consuming an array of fermented drinks for thousands of years. As mentioned earlier, they are nutritious and contain lots of vitamins, minerals, and enzymes. These lacto-fermented drinks have been made from fruits, milk, herbs, and grains. They possess medicinal qualities. Studies have indicated that these beverages are better at relieving thirst during bouts of physical labor because the minerals they contain replace those lost during perspiration. Additionally, when consumed with meals, they aid in digestion.[33] Fermented beverages are nature's soda.

Alcoholism is a problem that can be traced to nutritional deficiencies, particularly B vitamins and is an ever-growing problem in the United States. Our modern versions of beer and wine contain higher amounts of alcohol and a veritable cocktail of chemical additives, not to mention added sugar and genetically modified grains. That said, traditional cultures do imbibe in alcoholic beverages, in moderation; however, these beverages were simply fermented grapes, for instance, with no additives, no added sugars, and thus the alcohol content is lower. The same goes for beer in these cultures. Opt for organic wines and beers in moderation. Better yet, opt for lacto-fermented drinks that have health-giving properties.

Just Say No! to Soy

Soy contains very high levels of phytic acid and the usual process of soaking and sprouting does not neutralize the phytic acid; only very long periods of fermentation can effectively neutralize this layer. It is a known endocrine disruptor. Soy contains phytoestrogens that are detrimental to thyroid function. Trypsin inhibitors in soy inhibit the digestion of proteins. High heat processing of soy, such as is used in protein powders, denatures the proteins, and MSG is formed during this high heat processing; MSG is a known neurotoxin. Soy disrupts vitamin B pathways creating an imbalance and soy increases the body's need for vitamin D.[34]

Just say no to soy.

Pass the Butter, Please!

I know this may seem daunting and expensive, but it doesn't need to be. Making the switch to real food is, well, real simple. Finding a local farmers' market in your area is an important step; knowing your farmer has its perks! Honestly, my trip to the market each week is my favorite day of the week. I have grown to know and love each of these families. I love knowing that I am supporting them as they do what they love; and they do love what they do; and they do love talking with you about what they do! In many respects, they have become my friends. Find a market, even if it means going out of your way once a week. It is a great investment for your family and for your local community.

Real food is the ingredient, so to the extent possible, give up processed food-like products. They are expensive and not real food. Begin making your own condiments: ketchup, salad dressing, mayonnaise. Make bone broth regularly and use in soups and in cooking vegetables; make sure your bones are from pastured animals only (one more reason to find a local farmer.) Eggs from truly free-range chickens are a nutritional powerhouse and the yokes are an amazing vibrant shade of orange. Buying organic grains, legumes, and beans in bulk is a way of saving money. Planning ahead is key.

Use real butter from pastured cows. When preparing vegetables, always slather on the butter; the fat-soluble vitamins in the butter make the minerals and water-soluble vitamins in the vegetables bioavailable. See, there *is* a reason your grandmother used fats in her cooking! So, please pass the butter!

The journey of returning to a lifestyle of eating real, nutrient dense foods is one full of adventure and learning and good food. Enjoy the process! You deserve it!

10 | Tools for Your Toolbox

All disease begins in the gut
Hippocrates

*The human body heals itself and nutrition provides
the resources to accomplish this task.*
Roger Williams, Ph.D. (1971)

Shortly after my divorce, my daddy asked me what I wanted for Christmas. I told him I wanted a toolbox with tools (my husband had taken all of the tools with him, and rightly so, they were his) because one can't get by in life without the need for tools at one time or another. The need will surely arise for a flat-head screw driver, a Phillips-head screw driver, a hammer, a tape measure, pliers, or a wrench. So my daddy did just that: he bought me a bright yellow toolbox and filled it with all of the tools he thought I would need; I still have that toolbox and the tools!

Along with changing the type and quality of food you eat, there are other things to consider and other modalities that you can incorporate to improve and maintain your health.

Your Second Brain

Hippocrates said 2500 years ago that all disease begins in the gut. Now, research is proving him right and revealing that gut health is critical to overall health and that imbalances in the microbiome and the lining of the intestinal wall are the two variables that contribute to a host of diseases including diabetes, obesity, auto-immune diseases, heart disease, autism spectrum disorders, mood and behavioral disorders.

The enteric nervous system is located in the tissues lining the esophagus, stomach, small intestines, and colon. It is considered an entity unto its own and is considered the second brain; it is a network of neurons, neurotransmitters, and proteins that communicate together with a circuitry which enables it to act independently.

Almost every substance that operates in the brain is also present in the gut. Neurotransmitters such as serotonin, dopamine, and norepinephrine are also present in the gut. Proteins present in the brain are also present in the gut. The psychoactive chemical benzodiazepine is also present in the gut. It is a system unto itself; yet it communicates with the brain, or the central nervous system, through the vagus nerve.

Ever wonder why when you're anxious you get stomach upset? Or why you get "butterflies" when you are nervous? Or why you may "choke" with emotion? This is because what goes on in the "head" brain also affects the "gut" brain by way of the vagus nerve. This is why being under constant stress can have such a huge impact on your health.

Gut Flora

Our intestinal tract houses approximately 100 *trillion* microorganisms. In fact, our gut contains 10 times more bacteria than human cells, many of which are not yet fully identified; only about 400 different species have been identified so far. These microorganisms, or flora, play a large role in the function of the gut, provides protection from infection, regulates the metabolism, and comprises about 70-80% of our immune system. Ideally, there is a balance between the good flora (beneficial), the bad flora (pathogenic), and the commensal flora (neutral). The imbalance of these bacteria is linked to diseases ranging from depression to autoimmunity to Type 1 Diabetes, as well as neurological disorders, Alzheimer's, Parkinson's, multiple sclerosis, and autism.

As has been fully demonstrated, our lifestyle, diets high in refined carbohydrates and sugar and processed foods, the environmental toxins, and prescription medications, especially antibiotics, birth control, and stress are all culprits in disrupting the balance of the flora in our guts.

Gut Lining

The lining of our intestinal tract protects the body from the outside world. When things are working properly, substances that enter the mouth and which are not digested pass through to the other end and are eliminated. However, when this lining becomes permeable (leaky), meaning small holes appear in the lining, large proteins, particularly gliadin, the protein in gluten, and toxins can easily enter the blood stream. When that happens, because these substances do not belong there, the immune system does what it is designed to do and initiates an immune response and attacks the foreign substances. It is this immune response which creates inflammation.

Inflammation is not necessarily a bad thing. When you sprain your ankle and it swells, that is the immune system rushing to the rescue; it is normal and it is necessary. The problems begin when the immune system is constantly, daily, initiating an immune response which puts the body in a continual state of inflammation and the immune system begins attacking itself by attacking organs and tissues. It is this constant state of systemic internal inflammation that leads to disease.

The symptoms of leaky gut are not always digestive issues; leaky gut can also manifest in conditions such as psoriasis or eczema, rheumatoid arthritis or joint problems, heart disease, thyroid disease, depression, fibromyalgia, multiple sclerosis, asthma, irritable bowel syndrome, other digestive issues, and most other chronic and degenerative diseases.

Rebuild and Restore

While the conventional treatment for inflammation is the suppression of the immune system with anti-inflammatory medications and steroids, it fails to get to the root of the problem and that is a disruption in the integrity of the intestinal tract. There is no quick fix. Reducing the inflammation with medication does not correct the problem nor does it halt the underlying disease process. The *cause* of the inflammation must be addressed and turned off.

There are a myriad of factors that can cause the inflammatory response to get stuck in the "on" position, or in other words, disrupt the delicate balance and integrity of the digestive tract. Dr. David Marquis notes that it is important to evaluate causative factors that create an inflammatory environment:[1]

- Diet: alcohol, gluten, casein, processed foods, sugar, fast food
- Medications: corticosteroids, antibiotics, antacids, xenobiotics
- Infections: such as h-pylori, yeast and bacterial overgrowth, viral or parasite infections, Lyme, Epstein Barr virus
- Stress: increased cortisol, increased catecholamines
- Hormonal: thyroid, progesterone, estradiol, testosterone
- Neurological: brain trauma, stroke, neuro-degeneration
- Metabolic: glycosylated end products (inflammatory products of sugar metabolism), intestinal inflammation, autoimmune

Inflammation is a symptom pointing to a deeper, root cause and it is important to discover this cause for that is where true healing begins. This is also where the importance and quality of food matters, first as a cause and second as a way of restoring intestinal health.

Because many of our chronic diseases are autoimmune diseases and many of these autoimmune diseases are attributable to intestinal permeability (inflammatory response attacking various organs and tissues in the body), it is critical that you take the necessary steps to rebuild the lining of the intestinal wall and restore balance to the intestinal flora, both of which require a shift in what and how you eat and live.

GAPS

Dr. Natasha Campbell-McBride, a neurologist, neurosurgeon, and nutritionist created the GAPS Nutritional Protocol after her son was diagnosed with autism. Her book, *Gut and Psychology Syndrome* (GAPS), outlines the protocol she used to reverse her son's autism. She has since treated thousands of patients, both children and adults, suffering from learning disabilities, psychological disorders, digestive, and immune disorders. However, the book is a self-help book that describes the process in detail so that anyone can have access to this protocol.

Dr. Campbell-McBride created GAPS using the Specific Carbohydrate Diet (SCD) and modified it to emphasize traditional foods (see previous chapter), particularly meat stocks and bone broth. The diet is the most important part of the treatment which is rich and nutrient dense. She also incorporates supplements, but only a bare minimum. The final part of the protocol is lifestyle and detoxification. Removing offending toxins is an important part of healing and detoxification.

The GAPS protocol can be challenging, especially in the beginning stages where the first phase is focused solely on sealing the gut lining with healing broth. If you have serious compromises in your intestinal integrity, I highly recommend this protocol; it has proven effective many times over. While it is a self-help text, you may want the assistance of a naturopathic doctor or a health coach to walk with you through this process, particularly the introduction phase. GAPS is a longer-term protocol that can last from six months to two years, which makes sense. It takes years to get to the point of autoimmunity and other diseases; it is not something that can be fixed in the short term.

Autoimmune Paleo

The Autoimmune Paleo (AIP) diet is similar to GAPS, but has a much shorter duration and without the emphasis on traditional foods. It primarily consists of quality meats and vegetables, minimal frutis, and eliminates all grains, sugar, legumes, dairy, eggs, nightshades, processed foods, and alcohol. This protocol, also, can be very effective at restoring balance to the intestinal tract. It is generally followed for 30 days after which time a return to the regular paleo diet, slowly adding back some of the foods eliminated.

Paleo / Primal

Paleo is a prescribed way of eating that avoids all grains, legumes, dairy, refined sugar, white potatoes, processed foods, and refined oils. The focus is on consuming meats from pastured animals, fish/shellfish, fruits and vegetables, eggs, nuts and seeds, and healthy oils such as olive oil, avocado oil, and coconut oil. Primal is paleo, but it allows for a small amount of raw dairy. Fermented vegetables and fermented dairy are also enjoyed.

Wise Traditions Approach

The Weston A. Price Foundation (WAPF) is a foundation established to educate on the principles of eating based on traditional cultures as discovered by Dr. Price, or Wise Traditions. As outlined in the previous chapter, the major difference between the Wise Traditions approach and paleo is the inclusion of properly prepared soaked, sprouted, or fermented grains and raw and fermented dairy, and the use of healthy animal fats from pastured animals. The Wise Traditions approach focuses on incorporating nutrient dense foods into your diet, traditional preparation methods, and on pre-pregnancy nutrition and raising healthy children.

It should be noted that the grains of traditional cultures and the grains espoused for use by WAPF are not modern grains, but rather ancient grains such as einkorn, spelt, kamut, and teff.

WAPF does not advocate the use of modern grains. Modern wheat is extremely hybridized which has increased the gluten (gliadin) content of wheat making the amount of gluten exponentially higher than ancient wheat. Also, modern wheat is chemically engineered to resist herbicide, meaning it is sprayed with glyphosate containing herbicides before harvest; it is absorbed into the plant and it cannot be washed off and should be strictly avoided.

If, however, you need to heal your intestinal tract, avoiding grains altogether is an important consideration, while adhering to the remaining principles; that is also the basis of the GAPS protocol described above.

For children and young mothers and fathers, a diet rich in nutrient dense foods, healthy animal fats, and quality protein is absolutely essential for the health of the parents prior to conception, which ensures the health of the baby to be conceived. Within the principles of the Weston A. Price Foundation you will find the education you need on nourishing fertility and on nourishing children.

Vegetarian/Vegan

While there are times when one may want to restrict the intake of meat and animal products, such as times of cleansing which all cultures exercised, it is not ideal for the long term. And while certain plants do contain some proteins, plant proteins are not complete proteins, meaning they are missing an "essential" amino acid. Some contend that these missing nutrients can be supplemented; however, supplementation of isolated, synthetic compounds are not assimilated by the body. According to Dr. Campbell-McBride, "When Mother Nature designed the human body we weren't intended to get our nutrition from supplementation. All nutrients are supposed to come into our bodies holding hands with other nutrients. Only in that form can they be used properly by the body. No pill can provide that – only food."[2]

Vitamins and minerals work in tandem with one another, not as isolated constituents.

Those who adhere to a plant-based diet only will struggle and they will be left with nutritional deficiencies over time. Those of child-bearing age and young children, especially, should avoid a plant-based only diet. Fats from pastured animals supply much needed nutrients for brain and neurological development.

Beyond Food

Herbs, Herbals, and Herbalism

Just as our Creator gave us food as medicine, so He gave us herbs as medicine and He gave the ancients wisdom in how to use them. The earliest record of herbs being used dates back 5,000 years. This ancient art of healing has never gone out of use until the last 100 years in this country; it is still practiced heavily in other parts of the world. According to the World Health Organization (WHO) three-quarters of the globe's population relies on traditional medicines and of that use of traditional medicine, 85% comes from the use of plant medicine.[3]

However, there is a resurgence happening in the United Sates. Until the early 1900s, herbalism was a thriving practice with schools, textbooks, and trained practitioners; that is until the Rockefellers and the Carnegies bank-rolled the takeover of the medical profession by the American Medical Association.

With the new system came a new paradigm: one solution, one-size-fits-all-pop-a-pill paradigm. But that is not the tenet of ancient wisdom. In fact, the ancient art of healing took a holistic approach to health, incorporating the physical, emotional, and environmental. Each culture around the world had its own form of herbalism and use of medicinal plants. In the United States today, three major traditions co-exist: Ayurveda, Traditional Chinese Medicine, and the Western Herbal tradition. The wisdom of these ancient traditions can have a profound effect on your health, whether you have minor issues or full blown chronic inflammatory conditions.

Ayurveda

Ayurveda (āyur vēda) is a holistic system of medicine practiced in India which takes into consideration the mind, body, and spirit. In Sanskrit "Ayus" means "life" and "veda" means "deep knowledge or wisdom," so Ayurveda means the "wisdom of life" or "knowledge of longevity" and is based on a philosophy that we are all unique. It is a complete system of caring for health designed to promote a way of life, rather than the occasional treatment for illness. While Ayurveda has been around for 5,000 years, it is by no means primitive; it is quite complex and sophisticated.

Ayurveda recognizes that each person is unique and because of each individual's uniqueness, it offers a customizable approach. It operates off the principle of maintaining a state of balance and that each individual has an inherent state of balance which is unique to them; the opposite of the "one size fits all" paradigm. This balance involves the body, the mind, and the spirit and it teaches that balance should be maintained in order to achieve good health.

Ayurveda believes that each person has a constitution that is unique to the individual and moving away from that creates an imbalance and that the sign that one is moving away from balance is an alarm that something is amiss. It believes that the body has three primary types of constitution or *doshas*: *vata*, *pitta*, and *kapha*, which are made up of five different elements that manifest in the natural world. A person's constitution is made up of all three *doshas*; however, a person generally has a dominant *dosha*. To understand how to maintain balance, you must first know your dominant *dosha*, then you will know how to achieve and maintain balance.

This balance in the body is accomplished with food, spices, and herbs. For instance, if you tend to be a *vata*, you may be thin and run cold, you would include warming foods, spices, and herbs. Spices and herbs are an extension of our food and they are utilized every day by including them in meals and in teas; this is food as medicine. When necessary, they are included in larger amounts or in combination to provide stronger medicinal properties.

Ayurveda believes that when you are out of balance that you have committed crimes against wisdom and ceased to listen to your inner voice. Ayurveda includes several strategies to keep your *doshas* in balance:

- Keep the digestive fire (*agni)* strong; if digestion is compromised, so is health

- Food is the substance of life; celebrate your food and be present during meals

- Create a daily routine wherein you incorporate practices that bolster you and not detract from your health

- Maintain natural rhythms of life. In a world that constantly strives for a fountain of youth, embrace the place you are and keep with natural circadian rhythms.

As a tradition that has been around for thousands of years, there is much wisdom contained within its teachings which we can glean and apply in our own lives.

Traditional Chinese Medicine

Traditional Chinese Medicine (TCM) has been in existence for about 3,000 years. It is very similar to Ayurveda in principle: that of either being in balance or out of balance, the *yin* and *yang* must remain in balance with one another. You may be familiar with the symbol of yin and yang: a circle with one half black and one half white, with a small black circle within the white and a small white circle within the black; this represents balance.

Mistaken Fundamental Concepts of TCM
The prevalent belief is that we have a life force within us "Qi" (pronounced "chee"). This force is both physical and spiritual. This belief holds that we are born with a certain amount of Qi

which can never be added to, yet it can be depleted. Qi permeates the body and it informs the blood, nervous and lymphatic systems. It is protective from environmental forces such as viruses and it transforms the foods we eat into usable substances for the body. It regulates the body's temperature and facilitates movement and growth. TCM works with Qi to keep the body in balance by either unblocking the flow of Qi when it is blocked or by nourishing Qi if it is deficient.

While Qi is a life force within the body and present everywhere, it does have main pathways that carry it throughout the body. These pathways, or channels, are called meridians and they are bilateral, meaning they are on both sides of the body. There are 12 in all with six being more *yin*: and six being more *yang*. The six *yin* meridians, kidneys, spleen, heart, lungs, and pericardium, function to store vital "essences" of the body. The six *yang* meridians, bladder, gallbladder, stomach, small intestine, large intestine, and the "triple burner" which regulates body temperature, function to transport fluids and food. There are an additional six meridians: which run up the center of the body and up the spine.

Correct Fundamental Concepts of TCM

These prevalent beliefs about TCM have been difficult for western medicine to accept, and understandably so. The good news is that these mistaken beliefs are based on the incorrect translation of some terms in the Chinese medicine text *Huangdi Neijing* (HDNJ). Within the HDNJ, there are several sections; some dealing with anatomy and some dealing with pathology. Approximately 2500 years ago the Chinese were performing dissections, weighing and measuring internal organs, and describing their functions. Additionally, this text also described diseases, origins of the disease, and how to treat them with acupuncture, herbal medicine, dietary and lifestyle changes.[4]

The problem began when George Soulie de Morant, a French bank clerk, attempted to translate the Chinese text. One difficulty was his translation of the word Qi as "energy" when in fact the original Chinese word means oxygen. "In the *Huangdi*

Neijing, the Chinese describe the lungs breathing in what they call 'da qi.' If you look up da qi in a Chinese dictionary, you'll see it defined as 'great air.' The Chinese explained that the lungs breathed in air, and the lungs extracted the qi from the da qi."[5] Basically, qi does not mean energy, rather it is the concept of a "vital vapor" or the "essence of air." While the molecule known as oxygen had not yet been identified, the Chinese understood that something important was derived from the air that we breathe and they understood that this qi circulated throughout the body through the blood.

Another mistranslated word that has led to the mistaken concepts of TCM is the word "mai." Morant incorrectly translated this word to mean "meridian." The correct translation is "vessel" and "xue mai" is translated as blood vessel. There was no mysterious "energy" that was circulating through the equally enigmatic "meridians."[6]

Additionally, Morant translated the word "jie" as the "point" used in acupuncture. However, the more accurate translation of the word "jie" is "node, neurovascular node, or critical juncture." Current research has determined that these "nodes" contain "high concentrations of sensory fibers, fine blood vessels, fine lymphatic vessels, and mast cells."[7] What the Chinese understood is that these "nodes" which are on the surface of the body, can indicate disease in particular organs in the body and when these "nodes" are stimulated, it results in pain relief and resolution of problems with internal organs.[8]

> When the terms qi (oxygen), mai (vessel), and jie (neurovascular node) are properly translated, it becomes clear that there is no disagreement between ancient Chinese medical theory and contemporary principles of anatomy and physiology. Chinese medicine is not a metaphysical, energy medicine but instead a "flesh and bones" medicine concerned with the proper flow of oxygen and blood through the vascular system.[9]

As in Ayurveda, the use of many different medicinal plants with antiviral, antibacterial and immune-enhancing properties is foundational in TCM. Some formulas combine eight to twelve Chinese herbs in a capsule or as dried herbs to make a tea. TCM also employs the use of cupping, acupressure, and *qigong* which is a form of energetic movement and breathing techniques used to release the flow of qi; or in other words, to increase the amount of oxygen in the blood, which in turn, along with glucose, move through the cardiovascular system to produce energy through the Krebs cycle.

Like Ayurveda and all other cultures around the world, TCM also believes that each individual is unique and while two people may both suffer from the same illness, how they are treated for that illness will be different for each individual. Maintaining balance in the body and in life is crucial as is the use of spices and herbs for nutritional benefit as well as medicinal properties.

Western Herbalism

Western Herbalism, like Ayurveda and TCM, believes in the individual's uniqueness and that we each possess a certain constitution. While Ayurveda refers to this as *doshas* and TCM refers to it as *Qi* and the *yin/yang* balance, Western Herbalism uses the four humors: choleric, sanguine, melancholic, and phlegmatic, and the essence of energetics: hot/cold, dry/damp to describe the conditions in the body. Just as in Ayurveda, someone who tends to be cold would need more warming foods, spices, and herbs, so it is in Western Herbalism. This is the idea of matching the herbal therapies to the person rather than to a particular disease because the plants have the same energetics as people, hot/cold, dry/damp. If your general constitution is cold and dry and you begin to feel hot and damp (e.g. when you have a respiratory illness), then you can match the herbals to restore the balance and bring you back to your normal constitution of cold and dry.[10] Like Ayurveda and TCM, Western Herbalism believes that we have a dominate constitution.

Another piece in all three of these traditions is that of the taste of the herbs themselves. In TCM and Western Herbalism there are five tastes: pungent, salty, sour, bitter, and sweet. Ayurveda adds as sixth: astringent. Each of the different "tastes" of herbs represents the effect it will have on restoring balance to the body.

Ayurveda explains the process of how taste (*rasa*) works to promote balance in the body. It does this by breaking down the *rasa* into three separate parts: *rasa* (the initial taste), *virya* (warm versus cool), and *vipaka* (the post-digestive effect). The effect of food and herbs on the body after digestion can be described and viewed through this lens. *Rasa* and *virya* are fairly simple. Which of the six tastes is the food or herb and is the food or herb warming or cooling? The final component, *vipaka* is a little more complex in determining the effect on the body after digestion. There are two post-digestive effects: is the food or herb tonifying or is it purifying? To tone would be to strengthen and build up. Purifying foods and herbs would purify and remove tissue or toxins.[11]

As you can see, herbalism, in all of its forms, is not about prescribing "x" herb for "y" condition. Aren't you glad? I rather like that we can celebrate our individual uniqueness. It is important, however, that you know yourself and determine your normal constitution; but don't let that stop you from using herbs and spices liberally in your food daily.

God in his grace and mercy has given us food as medicine and herbs as medicine, and when used on a regular, daily basis in cooking, in teas, syrups, in tinctures and decoctions, they provide support to the immune system, the digestive system, and the nervous system. They are antimicrobial and they are powerful antioxidants. Their use as a part of life, daily, is another tool to strengthen the body.

If you are experiencing chronic health conditions, I encourage you to seek out practitioners of these healing arts; as well, most naturopathic doctors are also trained in these modalities and they have access to herbs that are not commonly grown in backyard gardens, but which possess incredible medicinal properties.

Homeopathy

Homeopathy, more than herbalism, has taken a beating from the allopathic medical system. It is hard to argue with the effectiveness of a system that has been around for 5,000 years with many pharmaceuticals based on plant constituents. Homeopathy in its present form, on the other hand, has only been in existence for approximately 225 years; however, its roots date back to Hippocrates.[12] Yet, it is a very effective treatment at the fraction of the cost of allopathic, prescription-driven medicine. Rockefeller himself used homeopathy and wanted the AMA to include their schools within the new model of medicine he was creating, but the doctors refused because it was not as profitable.[13]

Homeopathy is based on the principle that "like cures like" which means that any substance that can produce symptoms in a healthy person can also cure similar symptoms in a person who is sick. It is safe for everyone to use, including pregnant women, children, and the elderly. It was developed by a German physician and chemist, Samuel Hahnemann around 1790 and is based on three Principles:[14]

- The law of similars: a substance in large doses can produce symptoms of illness in a healthy person can cure similar symptoms in a sick person if used in minimal doses.

- Minimal dose: successive dilutions enhance the curative properties of a substance while eradicating the side effects. Only a minute dose is needed to help cure.

- Whole-person prescribing: symptoms, pain, and disease do not occur in isolation but are an overall reflection of the person – see the person as a whole.

Along with the three principles, there are three sets of rules that apply to effectiveness, the Laws of Cure:[15]

- A remedy starts healing from the top of the body and works downward.
- It starts from within the body, working outward, and from major to minor organs
- Symptoms clear up in reverse order to their manner of appearance.

As with traditional herbal medicine beliefs, homeopaths also believe that it is necessary to consider a person's constitution as well as their mental and emotional state and that any treatment should adjust for these findings so that overall health is achieved.

It is hard to break free from the propaganda of so many years and I, too, was skeptical of homeopathy until I was given a remedy by my naturopathic doctor and it worked! Effectively. Powerfully. Now I understand why it is another modality that the conventional medical system does not want us to use.

The process used to make homeopathic remedies is very precise. It involves creating a mother tincture with the substance being used for a specific condition. The mother tincture is then diluted to create different strengths. It is succussed (shaken) and potentized until nothing remains of the original substance. It is not understood exactly how this works, but this process creates an energetic frequency or imprint of the original substance in the solution. It is then prescribed based on the law of similar to treat a particular illness or condition.

One of the most extraordinary alternatives provided by homeopathy is that of homeopathic immunization or homeoprophylaxis and referred to as nosodes. It is an excellent alternative to vaccines. Nosodes are made from a killed form of the disease (e.g. measles) or animal, mineral, or vegetable products as the source substance. They are then succussed and potentized so there are no longer any of the original molecules from the disease left in the substance. What is left is the energetic imprint of that disease. When it is introduced into the body, it essentially educates the immune system so that it will recognize the disease if met in the future and it builds an appropriate immune response. It is safe and effective. There are none of the additives, mercury, aluminum, preservatives, or any of the other foreign substances found in vaccines.[16]

Homeopathy can also be used with animals. If you don't have a homeopath in your area, most naturopathic doctors can suggest remedies for you. One more tool for your toolkit. As with everything, quality does matter and your naturopath or a homeopath can point you in the right direction.

Essential Oils – Not Just for Hippies!

Unless you've been living under a rock for the last few years, you've likely heard about essential oils; they are all the rage now, with good reason, as they have medicinal properties and are powerful antioxidants. They are an important tool; however, there are some caveats, too.

Essential oils are volatile compounds that have been distilled from plant materials: leaves, stems, bark, root, seeds, flowers, and fruit. This distillation process concentrates these compounds and one drop is very powerful. The oils in plants protect the plant from insects, shield the plant from a harsh environment, and help the plant adapt to its surroundings. Essential oils can be used as first aid treatment, prevention, in personal care products, and in chemical free cleaning products. Many of the constituents in essential oils have antibacterial, antimicrobial, antifungal, antiviral, and antiseptic properties.

Though the use of essentials oils seems relatively new, they have, in fact, been in use for thousands of years dating back to ancient cultures in Greece, Rome, Egypt, China, and Israel. There are at least thirty-three different essential oils mentioned in the bible and more than a thousand references to their use, ranging from spiritual worship, to purification, to wellness.

The compounds in essential oils are unique molecular constituents that are readily absorbed into the bloodstream with the ability to pass through the blood-brain barrier. There are three ways to use essential oils: inhalation, topical, and oral.

Inhalation

Inhalation is by far the best and safest way to get essential oils into your system. And unless you are using for skin or muscular issues, inhalation is the most effective. As you inhale through the nasal passage, the olfactory nerve senses the aromatic and then it is absorbed into the brain where it has an effect on the brain cells and an effect on neurochemicals.

Topical

Topical use is beneficial for skin or muscle issues; however, essential oils should never be applied to the skin without first being diluted in a carrier oil. Carrier oils include fractionated coconut oil, jojoba oil, grapeseed oil, almond oil, and others. For skin care products, use butters such as shea and coca and other healthful options. Essential oils are an excellent alternative for skin care and household cleaning products. Replace your chemical-laden products with healthy ones.

Oral

There are several companies selling essential oils that promote the internal use of oils and though there may be times when this is beneficial, there are important caveats to keep in mind and some considerations and safety issues that need to be addressed.

I do not recommend the oral use of essential oils in the way that companies selling essential oils recommend them by placing a couple drops into a glass of water or in a veggie capsule. Remember, essential oils are volatile compounds and should never be used in the nose, eyes, or ears because of the fragile mucus membranes in those areas. The same holds true for the fragile mucus membranes in the mouth, esophagus, and stomach. Oil and water do not mix, so ingesting essential oils with water exposes the vulnerable membranes in the mouth, esophagus, and stomach to damage over the long term.

Additionally, these oils have antibacterial properties and ingesting them orally on a regular basis may disrupt that delicate flora in the intestinal tract over time. If taking for digestive upset, it is best to buy quality essential oils that are in enteric coated capsules, so that they will reach the digestive tract and then they should only be used for no longer than ten days. Ingesting them in water (or even diluted in fat such as coconut oil) will not ensure their transit to the intestinal tract. From the stomach they enter the bloodstream and are metabolized in the liver and then excreted through the kidneys. If you feel the need to use essential oils orally, please do so only under the guidance of a licensed aromatherapist or naturopathic doctor.

Essential Oil Quality Matters

It is important to make sure that the oils you are using are of high quality. Some companies claim their oils are "therapeutic" and in fact they are very concentrated and pure; however, they are not regulated and this label comes from the companies themselves. There are a number of variables that determine quality: climate, soil, and region where the plant is grown, and time of harvest all play a significant role in the amount and quality of the constituents in the oil. How the plant material is processed is also important. Steam-distilled and cold-pressed are the best methods for this truly leaves nothing but the essential oil. There is also a solvent-distilled method; however, this method leaves residue of the solvent in the oil and is best avoided.

It is important to do your research and learn about essential oils and different companies before investing in them. These oils are powerful and a little goes a long way. Some oils, especially the citrus oils, can be photosensitive, meaning use on the skin and going out in the sun or a tanning bed can cause damage to the skin. Also, care should be exercised when using with children. Some oils may be used on pets; while others are toxic to animals, especially cats. Educate yourself; this is an important step before using any oils.

It takes hundreds and sometimes thousands of pounds of plant material to get one pound of essential oil. They are precious compounds. Be judicious in your use of them. When stored properly, they have a long shelf-life. Keep in mind that they are not a substitute for dietary and lifestyle changes for your health; rather they are an adjunct. I see some companies promoting their use for anything and everything without making significant changes in diet; this is egregious and it is nothing more than substituting an oil for a pill. They are a very small piece, not the end-all-be-all solution to what ails you.

One last thought and consideration on essentials oils. They are powerful compounds with antibacterial, antiviral, antifungal, antimicrobial, antiseptic, and anti-inflammatory properties. As with anything *anti-* overuse could result in stronger and more virulent strains of these organisms. While there are those who posit that essential oils cannot cause resistance due to the complexity of these compounds, this could be a dangerous position to take because we simply do not know that for certain. Be judicious in your use of these amazing compounds so that they will remain viable tools for generations to come.

You Are Unique

You are fearfully and wonderfully made. Those 100 trillion microorganisms are uniquely yours; no one else has the exact same combination as you do. Your unique microbiome should contain a great diversity of organisms. A healthy diet full of pesticide free fruits and vegetables will feed those microorganisms and keep them diverse and functioning optimally. A diet with little fiber and processed foods will cause an imbalance which leads to chronic illness and degeneration. Restoring the balance is a critical piece in regaining health.

I love that these micro-organisms are referred to as flora; it speaks to the beauty and the bounty and the uniqueness that is *you*!

Your constitution is uniquely yours as well. Health and healing are possible; however, it will not come without changes to the status quo. And it will not come overnight if you are dealing with chronic conditions; however, it will come if you apply these principles. There is hope and healing to be attained.

11 | What's Life Got to Do With It?

If people only knew the healing power of laughter and joy,
many of our fine doctors would be out of business.
Joy is one of Nature's greatest medicines.
Joy is always healthy. A pleasant state of mind tends
to bring abnormal conditions back to normal.
Catherine Ponder

Do not be grieved, for the joy of the Lord is your strength.
Nehemiah 8:10b

What's life got to do with it? *(Cue Tina Turner's song.)* Only
everything! We live in a world where everything is compartmentalized. We separate our work life from our personal life from
our spiritual life from our physical health. But it is all connected.
We can't separate our mind from our body or our spirit from our
body. It is a beautiful whole.

You can eat healthy, but if there are imbalances in your life
and in your environment, your health will suffer. The wisdom of
the ancients has taught us this. How are your relationships? Are
you getting enough exercise? Are you getting adequate sleep? Do
you ever have fun or do you work, work, work all the time? Are
you taking care of you?

Stress as a Way of Life

The admonition to "reduce stress" is so commonplace that it has lost all meaning. Even so, it is imperative that we heed the admonition. I think it is fair to say that many people live under some form of chronic or persistent stress; a slow burn of accumulated stress-filled life situations from benign, fleeting frustrations, to malignant, enduring life-altering events. Unchecked, these will lead to serious health problems.

What happens in your body when you're under stress? The physiological stress response innate in all of us, the fight or flight response, prepares the body to face danger: the hypothalamus sends signals to the adrenals to release adrenaline and cortisol which is a good thing if you're trying to outrun a bear. This raises blood pressure, blood sugar, and provokes an immune response. This is necessary in the short term, but when the stress response is in a perpetual state of fight or flight and the adrenals are continually producing stress hormones it begins causing chronic inflammation.

Remember, too, the connection between the brain and the digestive tract. What is going on in our heads, will replay in our guts causing leaky gut and a disruption of the delicate flora that resides there. Because the gut also produces neurotransmitters such as dopamine, norepinephrine, and serotonin, these will also be altered and impact how we feel and impact our emotions.

Life happens. If you are living and breathing, you will encounter stressful situations. Often times, we bury the feelings we are experiencing as a result of the stress. It could be frustration, sadness, anger, fear, doubt, any number of negative emotions. It is okay to experience the gamut of emotions; it is when we repress these emotions that it becomes a problem; they are then stored in our bodies. It is easy to think that our emotions are separate from our bodies, but they are not.

The limbic system, which contains the hypothalamus, is considered the "seat of emotions" and there is constant communication and networking happening between the neurological system, endocrine system, and the immune system by way of neuropeptides. When we experience emotional trauma of any degree, neuropeptides are released and receptors throughout the body receive and store them.[1] This is why you could experience knee pain or back pain without having incurred a physical injury and no "cause" seems to exist.

That is how I ended up in the hospital all those years ago. While I did not understand it at the time and my doctor attributed it to "stress," it was much more than that; it was the constant onslaught of emotional trauma over years that eventually manifested itself into a condition which required medical attention. I believe "stress" is a woefully inadequate term used to describe a physiological process which takes place in the body as a result of recurring emotional trauma or duress, big and small, over time.

However it is described, stress or emotional duress, it creates a cascade of health problems: sleep disturbances, cravings, weight gain, heart disease, increased risk of stroke, skin rashes, digestive issues, depression, behavioral disorders, muscle aches, and compromised immune system. It is important to be diligent in taking steps necessary to relieve stress and to change your perception of stress. Here are a few suggestions:

- Exercise or go for walks, especially in nature.
- Engage in hobbies you love.
- Unplug from technology and social media.
- Make time for you; schedule it.
- Seek out the services of a therapist.
- Just say no to certain things; don't over-schedule your life.
- Eat foods that are nutrient dense.
- Spend time with those whom you can trust.
- Change how you perceive stress.
- Develop and practice an attitude of gratitude.
- Get a massage!

I can here you lamenting that it's not as simple as that. It is and it isn't. Being intentional in how we handle the stressors of life is critical. Changing the way we perceive stress is just one way of managing when life happens; it's called reframing. As an example, you lose your job. You have two options. You can begin to take on a negative self-image of yourself and of life. Or, you can reframe the incident and view it as an opportunity to follow a dream you've been harboring for years. Mindfulness is the key. Realizing that we can't control everything is crucial, so focus on what you can control and change the way you perceive the stressors of life.

I realize there are those who have endured horrific events and I am in no way down-playing those events; quite the opposite. It is a serious piece in your overall health. If you have experienced significant emotional trauma at any point in your life, particularly as a child, it is necessary to seek the assistance of a professional who can walk you through the process of releasing those emotions stored in the body.

Are You Getting Adequate Sleep?

Growing up we begged our parents to let us stay up just 10 more minutes. As adults, we hit the snooze in the morning because... *I just need 10 more minutes.* Or we brag that we can function on only 5 hours of sleep; eventually, the body will come to collect the debt. It is safe to say that most people are not getting enough sleep. Not only are we not getting enough sleep, but we're not getting enough restful sleep either.

According to the CDC, one in three adults reported getting less than 7 hours of sleep a night. Additionally, the CDC has declared insufficient sleep a public health problem, linking insufficient sleep to "...motor vehicle crashes, industrial disasters, and medical and other occupational errors. Unintentionally falling asleep, nodding off while driving, and having difficulty performing daily tasks because of sleepiness may contribute to these hazardous outcomes."[2] The CDC has stated that lack of sufficient sleep is linked to chronic diseases including high blood pressure, diabetes, depression, obesity, and cancer and that approximately 50-70 million adults suffer from problems with sleep disorders.[3]

If you're getting less than five hours of sleep per night, then your risk of heart disease, heart attack, and/or stroke is doubled. There is also a link between lack of sleep and diabetes, insulin resistance, and weight gain.[4] So, how much sleep is enough? Children ages 1-2 need 11-14 hours; preschoolers need 10-13 hours; children 6-13 need 9-11 hours; teenagers need 8-10 hours, and adults need 7-9 hours of sleep each night.[5]

Aside from an over-scheduled life, modern technology is a major contributor to sleep disturbances. The amount of light in the evening, especially exposure to blue light from bulbs and electronics, inhibits the production of melatonin which is needed for sleep. Electromagnetic radiation from your cell phone and WiFi can disturb natural sleep rhythms. This is especially problematic for teenagers even if they restrict their technology use to daylight hours. Sleep deprivation has an adverse, cumulative effect over time.

A review of sleep studies covering a 50-year period revealed that getting adequate sleep in your middle years was like making a deposit in your health in your later years; in other words, adequate sleep in middle age contributed to better mental acuity 28 years later. Conversely, not getting adequate sleep, accumulating over time, can cause brain shrinkage which cam negatively impact mental acuity in later years.[6]

Getting less than 7 hours of a sleep for one night can impact your ability to think clearly the next day, which can impact your problem solving abilities. As well, there is an impact on your genes and it can contribute to inflammation and weaken your immune system. Getting an extra hour of sleep at night has the reverse effect, a boost to your immune system.

Sleep is important. It seems that sleep is always one of the first things to go when life gets busy or we are stressed. It is important to make adjustments, where necessary, to support our natural circadian rhythm:

- Get plenty of bright light from sun exposure during the day; this is necessary for the pineal gland to produce melatonin. Getting 10-15 minutes of bright sunlight in the morning will help to reset your circadian rhythm. Try to spend time outdoors during the day.

- Avoiding watching television and using your computer and electronic devices after the sun goes down will promote the natural production of melatonin. When daylight savings time is in operation, you will need to avoid blue light earlier than sun down. Installing blue reduction apps on your electronic devices or wearing a pair of blue blocking glasses in the evening will aid in this if you need to use electronics.

- If possible, turn off your phone and WiFi when you go to bed so as to avoid interference from electromagnetic fields (EMFs).

- Keep your bedroom completely dark, if possible. If you need to have light, try to get a low-watt yellow or orange bulb.

- Avoid caffeine in the afternoon and evening hours.

- Create a routine around preparing for bed that you follow each evening.

- Keep the temperature in the room cool, below 70 degrees is best.

If you have hormone imbalances or blood sugar issues, these can also cause sleep disturbances and working to get those back in balance will have a profound effect on your sleep. Good sleep is important and making it a priority will go a long way to restoring and maintaining your health.

Exercise / Movement / Fun

You don't need me to tell you to exercise; I believe we all know this is an important part of a healthy lifestyle. However, I do want to offer a caveat. Be wise about it. High intensity workouts are not the best option for everyone. In fact, for those with hypothyroidism or adrenal insufficiency, this can further stress your body and wreck your health; burst training would be a good option. Make sure that the exercise you have chosen fits with your current state of health. Yoga and Pilates are excellent alternatives for those who need less intense workouts to begin, and you can never go wrong with walking. Just move, and start slow if you must, but get moving!

Have fun. Enjoy life, your family, your friends; celebrate those relationships by being present, both physically and emotionally. Make time for them and for the things you enjoy. Cultivate those relationships. Be intentional. Show grace. Forgive immediately. Offer mercy. Love unconditionally. Be kind, especially to yourself.

Spiritual Life

Without faith in the One Who created it all, there would be no real truth, goodness, and beauty to save the world as Dostoevsky so correctly predicted.

Rest, such a simple word, but oh, the complexity which surrounds it. We throw that word around all the time without giving any real thought to what it actually means and all that it encompasses. Certainly, it includes getting adequate sleep. It also includes taking time away from labor. Yet, it is so much more than that.

When I think of rest, I think of the person of Christ for He *IS* our rest. He invites us to partake of Himself (John 6:53-58); we are to "eat" and "drink" Him. In other words, we are to put on Christ and we are to participate in His divine nature. He is eternal life and to remain in Him is to receive His life. What we take in, whether what we think, what we eat and drink, or what we invest our time in, either nourishes us or it doesn't. When we partake of Christ, we are nourishing our minds and our spirit.

Christ is the One in whom all things hold together and through whom God is revealed as the infinite fountain of love (Colossians 1:16-20). If all things are by Him, through Him, and for Him, then Truth, Goodness, and Beauty have their origins in the Triune. Truth is a person. Goodness is a Person. Beauty is a Person. And that Person is Christ.

Secularism and the Age of Enlightenment have taught us that knowledge is limited to what can be verified by empirical methods. We are bombarded every day with the world's view of "truth is relative," "goodness is morally relative," and "beauty is in the eye of the beholder" (who sees truth as relative). But truth, in fact, is rooted and has its origin in a Person as do goodness and beauty.

The Greek word for "beauty" is *kallos*, and the verb which is etymologically related to that is *kalein* which means "to call." Beauty, then, is an invitation to encounter a world filled with awe and wonder and to cultivate a life that embodies Truth, Goodness, and Beauty; this begins with worship (John 4:23-24). It is an invitation to living life nourished, seeking truth and goodness and beauty. Truth feeds the mind; Goodness nurtures the spirit; Beauty heals the soul.

Maybe it's just me. Maybe I just need it more, but I long for times of resting in beauty, whether that is music that stirs my soul on a deep level, or whether that is the written words of deep Christian thinkers who explore the vastness of our Christ, or whether that is the beauty of the natural world that surrounds us; I need it! Often! And so do you!

"Finally, brethren, whatever is true, whatever is honorable, whatever is right, whatever is pure, whatever is lovely, whatever is of good repute, if there is any excellence and if anything worthy of praise, dwell on those things." Philippians 4:8

With all that life throws at us each day; the hustle and bustle of living; the injustice that abounds in the world; the plethora of secularism with which we are affronted all day, every day; the hurts we endure – fill in the blank with you particular circumstance – we need to be intentional about seeking time to bind the wounds caused by it all, to bask in Truth, Goodness, and Beauty. It is healing. It is renewing. It is life.

I invite you to find and to pursue those things that stir your soul; those things that ignite awe and wonder and worship of the One who created it all. The enemy of your soul does not want you to live in awe and wonder; rather he wants you trapped in busyness (even busyness that appears good), and trapped by the entanglements of the world. Take care of you. Take care of your soul, so you can take care of those you love and serve. You can't pour from an empty cup.

Wholeness

Taking care of ourselves and our families goes beyond the foods we eat; while that is an important piece, it is only a piece and not the sole arbiter of true health. Correcting the imbalances in our personal lives is necessary also. Those who have gone before us thousands of years ago knew well the necessity of feeding your spirit as well as your body.

Do our children need to play every sport conceivable and participate in every extra-curricular activity? What has happened to the idea of doing one thing and doing it really well? I realize this is an unpopular idea; but it is possible to stretch ourselves and our children too thin. I am asking you to consider the pace at which you live life. It is okay to say no. I realize how hard that is; I was one of those people who said yes to everything and everyone and I learned the hard way that it's just not possible to be all things to all people all of the time.

Realize that not only are you what you eat, but you are also what you think. What we think, how we think, whether those thoughts are positive or negative, will have a physical effect on the body. Again, be kind to yourself.

We have all been placed here for a reason; take time to find out what your purpose is in life and make wholeness a priority rather than an afterthought.

12 | You've Got Wings, Baby!

It is not... that some people do not know
what to do with truth when it is offered to them,
but the tragic fate is to reach,
after patient search, a condition of mind-blindness in which
the truth is not recognized, though it stares you in the face."
Sir William Osler

I'm trying to free your mind, Neo.
But I can only show you the door.
You're the one that has to walk through it.
Morpheous, *The Matrix*

It's no use going back to yesterday,
because I was a different person then.
Alice, *Alice in Wonderland*

Congratulations on making it through to the other end of the rabbit hole and into the light of hope! For many of you, I know this has been a tremendous amount of information to absorb and perhaps you are feeling overwhelmed and wondering where to start. The answer to that will be different for each of you.

There was a time when I didn't know these truths; but when I learned them, it completely changed my life. I remember those early days when I began my research and I was uncovering information I had never heard, the truths contained here, and

I remember being stunned by it; so much so, that I knew I had to share it with you. I remember feeling guilty for not knowing and I remember thinking, *How did I not know this?* Rather than beat myself up because I felt like I should have known, I let the past stay in the past and moved forward with my new-found knowledge into a new-found way of living. We can't undo the past, but we can make better decisions and choices for the future going forward. We must!

Scripture directs us to be good stewards of our bodies and that includes the foods we eat as well as other substances we allow in our bodies and those of our children. It is a privilege which has been bestowed upon us to nourish our families and to protect our families and to be good stewards of the animals and of this planet which God has entrusted to our care.

I pray that you are not indifferent to the things that are going on behind the scenes and that you are not deceived by those who have a vested interest in making sure you continue to buy their poisons. In the words of Edmund Burke, "The only thing necessary for the triumph of evil is for good men to do nothing."

I cannot stress enough how important it is to be vigilant about what goes in your body and that of your family from food, to medications, to vaccines, to the products you use in your home and on your body. The choices you make today will directly impact the health of future generations. Heed the warning of Dr. Price 80 years ago: "The complacency with which the masses of the people as well as the politicians view our trend is not unlike the drifting of a merry party in the rapids above a great cataract. There seems to be no appropriate sense of impending doom."[1] Take note of the transgenerational epigenetic nature of continuing to live with a toxic burden on the generations still yet unborn.

We need to leave this world a better place than how we found it so that the next generation has a fighting chance. If we don't change the state of our food supply and medical system and maintain the most basic freedom of the right to decide what is best for our bodies and for our families, we have failed the next generation. What is the legacy that we are leaving them? As much as we may like to, we can't walk around with our head stuck in the sand or look the other way; by so doing, we are just as culpable. Remember, our food has been engineered to make us addicted and complacent. It takes courage to stand against popular opinion.

We must take responsibility for our actions; while we may not be able to control the food system, we can control what we choose to purchase. Make finding quality food a priority. We are to honor God and we are to bring Him glory. We think what we put into our bodies is separate and apart from our spiritual lives, but it is not. St. Ignatius of Loyola said, "The glory of God is man fully alive." But we are not fully alive; and while he was referring to the heart and soul of man, I posit that the health of our bodies is just as important as the health of our soul, especially when the foods we eat are engineered to dull our minds.

I pray that we will no longer remain complacent and complicit. We have a responsibility to future generations. It is up to us in the here and now to ensure their future. May we not be indifferent. We have abdicated the care of our families to the government, a/k/a career politicians, and to billion dollar corporations that are only concerned with lining their pockets. I love the way Natasha Campbell-McBride describes how we came to this place:

> For millennia it was the role of the women to look after their family's health. How did they do that? Through food. Women had sacred knowledge about what foods are good for what health problem and situation in life and this knowledge was passed from mother to daughter, from grandmother to granddaughter. But since humanity created the food industry, women relinquished their sacred power of looking after their families' health. Of course, the food industry's agenda is profit, not the health of your family.[2]

I pray that we, as a people, will reclaim our sacred, God-given responsibility to nourish our families as He intended. It is a privilege, really, this sacred responsibility. And while I have been referring to women as the primary nurturers of the family, I realize that men are also in that role, whether by design or because life happened and made it so. This is for you, too. It is for all of humanity.

In many respects, we have become a society of people who shirk any accountability for our own actions. This must stop if we are to ensure that future generations are healthy and well. This issue of what has been done to our food and our medical system is just too important to remain indifferent.

Once you know truth, you can't unknow it. Once you know truth, you have a moral obligation and a moral imperative to apply and to share that truth; there is a responsibility associated with it. There is an accountability associated with it. You have been informed. What are you going to do with it?

You've got wings, now! You are armed with truth! Use it!

Beloved, I pray that in all respects you may prosper and be in good health, just as your soul prospers.
3 John 1:2

Appendix "A"

Derivatives of GM Crops

Ascorbic acid

Baking powder

Calcium

Canola oil

Cellulose

Citric acid

Citrus cloud emulsion

Corn flour

Corn masa

Corn meal

Corn oil

Corn sugar

Corn syrup

Cornstarch

Cottonseed oil

Dextrin

Dextrose

Diglycerides

Ethel acetate

Ethylene

Ethyl lactate

Fibersol-2

Fructose

Fumaric Acid

Glucose

Gluten

High fructose corn syrup

Hydrolized vegetable protein

Inositol

Maltodextrin

Margarine	Soy sauce
Polydextrose	Starch
Protein isolate	Stearate
Saccharin	Sucrose
Semolina	Sugar (except cane)
Sorbic acid	Tamari
Sorbitol	Tocopherals (Vit. E)
Soy flour	Tofu
Soy isolates	Vanilla extract
Soy lecithin	Vegetable fats
Soy milk	Vegetable oils
Soy oil	White vinegar
Soy protein	Xanthum gum
Soy protein isolate	Xylitol

Appendix "B"

Hippocratic Oaths

(Original Version)

"I SWEAR by Apollo the physician, Aesculapius, and Health, and All-heal, and all the gods and goddesses, that, according to my ability and judgement, I will keep this Oath and this stipulation.

TO RECHON him who taught me this Art equally dear to me as my parents, to share my substance with him, and relieve his necessities if required; to look up his offspring in the same footing as my own brothers, and to teach them this art, if they shall wish to learn it, without fee or stipulation; and that by precept, lecture, and every other mode of instruction, I will impart a knowledge of the Art to my own sons, and those of my teachers, and to disciples bound by a stipulation and oath according the law of medicine, but to none others.

I WILL FOLLOW that system of regimen which, according to my ability and judgment, I consider for the benefit of my patients, and abstain from whatever is deleterious and mischievous. I will give no deadly medicine to any one if asked, nor suggest any such counsel; and in like manner I will not give a woman a pessary to produce abortion.

WITH PURITY AND WITH HOLINESS I will pass my life and practice my Art. I will not cut persons laboring under the stone, but will leave this to be done by men who are practitioners of this work. Into whatever houses I enter, I will go into them for the benefit of the sick, and will abstain from every voluntary act of mischief and corruption; and, further from the seduction of females or males, of freemen and slaves.

WHATEVER, IN CONNECTION with my professional practice or not, in connection with it, I see or hear, in the life of men, which ought not to be spoken of abroad, I will not divulge, as reckoning that all such should be kept secret.

WHILE I CONTINUE to keep this Oath unviolated, may it be granted to me to enjoy life and the practice of the art, respected by all men, in all times! But should I trespass and violate this Oath, may the reverse be my lot!"

* * *

(Modern Version)

I SWEAR in the presence of the Almighty and before my family, my teachers and my peers that according to my ability and judgment I will keep this Oath and Stipulation.

TO RECKON all who have taught me this art equally dear to me as my parents and in the same spirit and dedication to impart a knowledge of the art of medicine to others. I will continue with diligence to keep abreast of advances in medicine. I will treat without exception all who seek my ministrations, so long as the treatment of others is not compromised thereby, and I will seek the counsel of particularly skilled physicians where indicated for the benefit of my patient.

I WILL FOLLOW that method of treatment which according to my ability and judgment, I consider for the benefit of my patient and abstain from whatever is harmful or mischievous. I will neither prescribe nor administer a lethal dose of medicine to any patient even if asked nor counsel any such thing nor perform the utmost respect for every human life from fertilization to natural death and reject abortion that deliberately takes a unique human life.

WITH PURITY, HOLINESS AND BENEFICENCE I will pass my life and practice my art. Except for the prudent correction of an imminent danger, I will neither treat any patient nor carry out any research on any human being without the valid informed consent of the subject or the appropriate legal protector thereof, understanding that research must have as its purpose the furtherance of the health of that individual. Into whatever patient setting I enter, I will go for the benefit of the sick and will abstain from every voluntary act of mischief or corruption and further from the seduction of any patient.

WHATEVER IN CONNECTION with my professional practice or not in connection with it I may see or hear in the lives of my patients which ought not be spoken abroad, I will not divulge, reckoning that all such should be kept secret.

WHILE I CONTINUE to keep this Oath unviolated may it be granted to me to enjoy life and the practice of the art and science of medicine with the blessing of the Almighty and respected by my peers and society, but should I trespass and violate this Oath, may the reverse by my lot."

Demand that violations of this code be brought to light and those that insist on violationing it be prosecuted or minimally be made to resign from practice.

You will see on this website that the majority of psychiatric crimes are simple violations of this code.

Appendix "C"

Excerpts from Elie Wisel's speech
"Perils of Indifference" April 12, 1999

"What is indifference? A strange and unnatural state in which the lines blur between light and darkness, dusk and dawn, crime and punishment, cruelty and compassion, good and evil.

What are its courses and inescapable consequences? Is it a philosophy? Is there a philosophy of indifference conceivable? Can one possibly view indifference as a virtue? Is it necessary at times to practice it simply to keep one's sanity, live normally, enjoy a fine meal and a glass of wine, as the world around us experiences harrowing upheavals?

Of course, indifference can be tempting – more than that, seductive. It is so much easier to look away from victims. It is so much easier to avoid such rude interruptions to our work, our dreams, our hopes. It is, after all, awkward, troublesome, to be involved in another person's pain and despair. Yet, for the person who is indifferent, his or her neighbor are of no consequence. And, therefore, their lives are meaningless. Their hidden or even visible anguish is of no interest. Indifference reduces the other to an abstraction.

* * *

Rooted in our tradition, some of us felt that to be abandoned by humanity then was not the ultimate. We felt that to be abandoned by God was worse than to be punished by Him. Better an unjust God than an indifferent one. For us to be ignored by God was a harsher punishment than to be a victim of His anger. Man can live far from God – not outside God. God is wherever we are. Even in suffering? Even in suffering.

In a way, to be indifferent to that suffering is what makes the human being inhuman. Indifference, after all, is more dangerous than anger and hatred. Anger can at times be creative. One writes a great poem, a great symphony, one does something special for the sake of humanity because one is angry at the injustice that one witnesses. But indifference is never creative. Even hatred at times may elicit a response. You fight it. You denounce it. You disarm it. Indifference elicits no response. Indifference is not a response.

Indifference is not a beginning, it is an end. And, therefore, indifference is always the friend of the enemy, for it benefits the aggressor – never his victim, whose pain is magnified when he or she feels forgotten. The political prisoner in his cell, the hungry children, the homeless refugees – not to respond to their plight, not to relieve their solitude by offering them a spark of hope is to exile them from human memory. And in denying their humanity we betray our own.

Indifferent, then is not only a sin, it is a punishment. And this is one of the most important lessons of this outgoing century's wide-ranging experiments in good and evil.

In the place that I come from, society was composed of three simple categories: the killers, the victims, and the bystanders. During the darkest of times, inside the ghettos and death camps . . . we felt abandoned, forgotten. All of us did.

And our only miserable consolation was that we believed that Auschwitz and Treblinka were closely guarded secrets; that the leaders of the free world did not know what was going on behind those black gates and barbed wire; that they had no knowledge of the war against the Jews that Hitler's armies and their accomplices waged as part of the war against the Allies.

If they knew, we thought, surely those leaders would have moved heaven and earth to intervene. They would have spoken out with great outrage and conviction. They would have bombed the railways leading to Birkenau, just the railways, just once.

And now we knew, we learned, we discovered that the Pentagon knew, the State Department knew. And the illustrious occupant of the White House then, who was a great leader.

*　*　*

No doubt, he was a great leader. . . . why didn't he allow those refugees to embark . . . Why the indifference, on the highest level, to the suffering of the victims?

But then, there were human beings who were sensitive to our tragedy. Those non-Jews, those Christians, that we called the "Righteous Gentiles," whose selfless acts of heroism saved the honor of their faith. Why were there so few? Why was there a greater effort to save SS murderers after the war than to save their victims during the war?

Why did some of America's largest corporations continue to do business with Hitler's Germany... It has been suggested, and it was documented, that the Wehrmacht could not have conducted its invasion of France without oil obtained from American sources. How is one to explain their indifference?

*　*　*

Does it mean that we have learned from the past? Does it mean that society has changed? Has the human being become less indifferent and more human? Have we really learned from our experiences? Are we less insensitive to the plight of victims...?"

Resources

Books

Genetic Roulette
Jeffrey M. Smith

Altered Genes, Twisted Truth
Steven M. Druker

Poison Spring: The Secret History of Pollution and the EPA
E.G. Vallianatos

*CAFO (Concentrated Animal Feeding Operation):
The Tragedy of Industrial Animal Factories*
Edited by Daniel Imhoff

The Truth About Cancer
Ty M. Bollinger

Overdosed America: The Broken Promise of American Medicine
John Abramson, M.D.

Food Forensics
Mike Adams

Nourishing Traditions
Sally Fallon Morell

Gut and Psychology Syndrome
Natasha Campbell-McBride, M.D.

Nutrition and Physical Degeneration
Weston A. Price, DDS

Nourishing Broth
Sally Fallon Morell with Kaayla T. Daniel

Websites

Polyfacefarms.com
Joel Salatin, books and resources on sustainable farming

EWG.org
Environmental Working Group – information on chemicals in products and in the environment.

TheTruthAboutCancer.com

Vactruth.com
Independent information on vaccines

Responsibletechnology.org
Jeffrey Smith's organization, Institute for Responsible Technology
Information on GMOs

Sustainabletable.org
Education on sustainable local food and agriculture

Worldmercuryproject.org
Robert F. Kennedy, Jr.'s organization
Education and advocacy

Organicconsumers.org
Education and advocacy

Westonaprice.org
Foundation committed to education and advocacy for traditional
foods and preparation methods
Source raw milk

Realmilk.com
Education and advocacy for real (raw) milk

Culturesforhealth.com
Cultures and equipment for soaking, sprouting, fermenting

Heirloom Seed Saver Sites

Rareseeds.com
Baker Creek Heirloom Seeds

Seedsavers.org
Seed Savers Exchange

Southernexposure.com
Southern Exposure Seed Exchange

Endnotes

Chapter 1

1 Weston A. Price, DDS. *Nutrition and Physical Degeneration.* (Lemon Grove, CA: Price-Pottenger Nutrition Foundation: 1939/2014)

2 Weston A. Price, DDS. *Nutrition and Physical Degeneration.* (Lemon Grove, CA: Price-Pottenger Nutrition Foundation: 1939/2014), 368

3 RMIT University. "Sins of the father could weigh on the next generation." ScienceDaily. www.sciencedaily.com/releases/2015/12/151201113925.htm

4 Qi Chen, et cl., "Sperm tsRNAs contribute to intergenerational inheritance of an acquired metabolic disorder," *Science*, http://science.sciencemag.org/content/early/2015/12/29/science.aad7977.full, December 31, 2015, DOI: 10.1126/science

5 Weston A. Price, DDS, *Nutrition and Physical Degeneration.* (Lemon Grove, CA: Price-Pottenger Nutrition Foundation: 1939/2014), 355

6 Ibid., 321

Chapter 2

1 Palm Oil, What's the Issue? http://www.saynotopalmoil.com/Whats_the_issue.php

2 Lenoir M, Serre F, Cantin L, Ahmed SH (2007) "Intense Sweetness Surpasses Cocaine Reward," PLoS ONE 2(8): e698. doi:10.1371/journal.pone.0000698

3   Schulte EM, Avena NM, Gearhardt AN (2015) Which Foods May Be Addictive? The Roles of Processing, Fat Content, and Glycemic Load. PLoS ONE 10(2): e0117959, doi:10.1371/journal.pone.0117959

4   Joseph Mercola, DO, "Sugar Industry Secrets Exposed" (2015), http://articles.mercola.com/sites/articles/archive/2015/07/25/sugar-industry-secrets.aspx

5   Morley Safer, "The Flavorists: Tweaking tastes and creating cravings," 60 Minutes, CBS News, November 27, 2011, http://www.cbsnews.com/news/the-flavorists-tweaking-tastes-and-creating-cravings-27-11-2011/ and https://www.youtube.com/watch?v=a7Wh3uq1yTc

6   Tuula Tuormaa, "The adverse effects of food additives on health: a review of the literature with a special emphasis on childhood hyperactivity." Journal of Orthomolecular Medicine 9 (1994): 225-225.

7   Josh Axe, DNM, DC, CNS, *Eat Dirt* (New York, New York: Harper Collins, 2016)

8   Natasha Campbell-McBride, MD, "The Gut: Key to Good Health," Wise Traditions Podcast #5, https://www.westonaprice.org/uncategorized/wise-traditions-podcast/

9   Blaisdell AP, Lau YL, Telminova E, Lim HC, Fan B, Fast, CD, Garlick D, Pendergrass DC. "Food Quality and motivation: A refined low fat diet induces obesity and impairs performance on a progressive ratio schedule of instrumental lever pressing in rats," PhysiolBehav. 2014 Apr 10; 128:220-225. doi.10.1016/physbeh. s014.02.025. Epub 2014 Feb 16

Chapter 3

1   "Our Dwindling Food Variety," National Geographic, http://ngm.nationalgeographic.com/2011/07/food-ark/food-variety-graphic

2   "Seed Giants vs. U.S. Farmers," A Report by the Center for Food Safety and Save our Seeds. 2013. http://www.centerforfoodsafety.org/files/seed-giants_final_04424.pdf

3   Ibid.

4   Ibid.

5   M. Sean Kaminsky, "Open Sesame: The Story of Seeds," Film, directed by M. Sean Kaminsky, (2015, Open Pollinated Productions, LLC), DVD.

6   Ibid.

7   Unless otherwise noted, the information in this and following sections is sourced from Jeffrey M. Smith's book *Genetic Roulette* (Fairfield, IA: Yes! Books, 2007) and from his organization website Institute for Responsible Technology and from the speaker training I received on GMOs through the Institute of Responsible Technology. Jeffrey M. Smith is the foremost authority on genetically engineered and genetically modified organisms.

8   Carolann Wright, "Virtually indestructible rogue GMO grass threatens environment, wildlilfe, and industry," *The Event Chronicle*, June 14, 2017, http://www.theeventchronicle.com/news/north-america/virtually-indestructible-rogue-gmo-grass-threatens-environment-wildlife-industry/#

9   Medical Officer's Summary of Consultation, Meeting Symopsis, and Final Comments. http://www.biointegrity.org/FDAdocs/15/mlbbp.pdf

10 Jonathan Latham, "The Puppetmasters of Academia (or what the NY Times left out)," *Independent Science News*, Sept. 8, 2015. https://www.independentsciencenews.org/science-media/the-puppetmasters-of-academia-ny-times-left-out/

11 Steven M. Druker, *Altered Genes, Twisted Truth*, (Salt Lake City, UT: Clear River Press, 2015).

12 Danny Hakim, "Monsanto Weed Killer Roundup Faces New Doubts on Safety in Unsealed Documents," New York Times, March 14, 2017. https://www.nytimes.com/2017/03/14/business/monsanto-roundup-safety-lawsuit.html

13 *Seed: The Untold Story*, Film, Taggart Siegel and Jon Betz (2016, Collective Eye Films), DVD.

14 Marion Copley March 4, 2013 letter to Jess Rowland entered into court record. https://www.organicconsumers.org/sites/default/files/marioncopleyletter.pdf

15 Ibid.

16 Carey Gillam, "USDA drops plans to test for Monsanto weed killer in food," *U.S. Right to Know,* March 24, 2017. https://usrtk.org/pesticides/usda-drops-plan-to-test-for-monsanto-weed-killer-in-food/

17 "Correlation Of Rising Incidence Of Diseases And Chronic Health Conditions With GMOs And Glyphosate," *Institute for Responsible Technology,* http://responsibletechnology.org/correlation-of-rising-incidence-of-diseases-and-chronic-health-conditions-with-gmos-and-glyphosate-3/

Chapter 4

1 Joel Salatin. *Folks, this ain't normal: A Farmer's Advice for Happier Hens, Healthier People, and a Better World,* (New York, New York: Hachette Book Group, 2011)

2 Daniel Imhoff, *CAFO (Concentrated Animal Feeding Operation): The Tragedy of Industrial Animal Factories,* (Sausalito, CA: Foundation for Deep Ecology, 2010), xi

3 Unless otherwise noted, all information in the remainder of this chapter comes from *CAFO (Concentrated Animal Feeding Operation): The Tragedy of Industrial Animal Factories,* (Sausalito, CA: Foundation for Deep Ecology, 2010)

4 Ibid., 61

5 Ibid., 35

6 Carrie Hribar, "Understanding Concentrated Animal Feeding Operations and Their Impact on Communities," (Bowling Green, Oh: National Association of Local Boards of Health, 2010), 9

7 Fact Sheet: "Antibiotics and Industrial Farming 101," *The PEW Charitable Trusts,* May 5, 2014. http://www.pewtrusts.org/en/research-and-analysis/fact-sheets/2014/05/05/antibiotics-and-industrial-farming-101

Chapter 5

1 McManis, Vanessa. "Johns Hopkins study suggests medical errors are third-leading cause of death in U.S." May 3, 2016. https://hub.jhu.edu/2016/05/03/medical-errors-third-leading-cause-of-death/

2   Gary Null, "Death by Medicine," Organic Consumers Association http://www.webdc.com/pdfs/deathbymedicine.pdf

3   Ty M. Bollinger, *The Truth About Cancer: What You Need to Know About Cancer's History, Treatment, and Prevention*, (Hay House, Inc., 2016).

4   Ibid.

5   Ibid.

6   Ibid.

7   Ibid.

8   E. Richard Brown, *Rockefeller Medicine Men: Medicine and Capitalism in America*, (Lost Angeles, CA: University of California Press, 1979).

9   Ibid.

10   Ibid., 67

11   Ibid.

12   Ibid., 74

13   Ibid.

14   Ty M. Bollinger, *The Truth About Cancer: What You Need to Know About Cancer's History, Treatment, and Prevention*, (Hay House, Inc., 2016), 22

15   E. Richard Brown, *Rockefeller Medicine Men: Medicine and Capitalism in America*, (Lost Angeles, CA: University of California Press, 1979).

16   Ty M. Bollinger, *The Truth About Cancer: What You Need to Know About Cancer's History, Treatment, and Prevention*, (Hay House, Inc., 2016).

17   Daniel F. Weisberg, "Science in the Service of Patients: Lessons from the Past in the Moral Battle for the Future of Medical Education," *Yale Journal of Biology and Medicine*, 87 (2014) p. 79-89, p. 81

18   Thomas P. Duffy, "The Flexner Report – 100 Years Later," *Yale Journal of Biology and Medicine*, (2011), pp. 269-276.

19   Ibid., 274

20   Gabriel Donohoe, "Nuremberg Trials: Big Pharma's Crimes Against Humanity," *Natural News*, October 18, 2008, http://www.naturalnews.com/z024534_Europe_health_WHO.html

21 Mathhias Rath, "IG Farben and the History of the 'Business With Disease,'" Dr. Rath Health Foundation, http://www4.dr-rath-foundation.org/PHARMACEUTICAL_BUSINESS/history_of_the_pharmaceutical_industry.htm

22 Ibid.

23 Ty M. Bollinger, *The Truth About Cancer: What You Need to Know About Cancer's History, Treatment, and Prevention*, (Hay House, Inc., 2016), and E. Richard Brown, *Rockefeller Medicine Men: Medicine and Capitalism in America*, (Lost Angeles, CA: University of California Press, 1979).

24 Daniel F. Weisberg, "Science in the Service of Patients: Lessons from the Past in the Moral Battle for the Future of Medical Education," *Yale Journal of Biology and Medicine*, 87 (2014) p. 79-89, p. 87

25 Jim Marrs, *The Rise of the Fourth Reich: The Secret Societies that Threaten to Take Over America*, (New York NY: Harper Collins, 2008).

26 *Doctored*, Film, Directed by Bobby Sheehan (2012, Jeff Hays Films, Working Films). DVD

27 Aimee Picchi, "Drug ads: $5.2 billion annually -- and rising," CBSNews.com, March 11, 2016. http://www.cbsnews.com/news/drug-ads-5-2-billion-annually-and-rising/

28 Ibid.

29 Michelle Cortez, "Prescription Drug Spending Hits Record $425 Billion in U.S," *Bloomberg*, April 14, 2016. https://www.bloomberg.com/news/articles/2016-04-14/prescription-drug-spending-hits-record-425-billion-in-u-s

30 "Prescription Drugs: 7 Out Of 10 Americans Take At Least One, Study Finds," *Huffington Post*, June 19, 2013. http://www.huffingtonpost.com/2013/06/19/prescription-drugs-prevalence-americans_n_3466801.html

31 Gregory Smith, *American Addict*, Film, Sasha Knezev (2013, Pain MD Productions and 888 Films). DVD.

32 John Abramson, *Overdosed America*, (New York, NY: Harper Collins, 2008) 149

33 Healthcare Overhaul, *Center for Responsive Politics.*, OpenSecrets. org, https://www.opensecrets.org/news/issues/healthcare?type=A

34 "Pharma lobbying held deep influence over opioid policies," *The Center for Public Integrity*, https://www.publicintegrity.org/2016/09/18/20203/pharma-lobbying-held-deep-influence-over-opioid-policies

35 Gregory Smith, *American Addict*, Film, Sasha Knezev (2013, Pain MD Productions and 888 Films). DVD.

36 John Abramson, *Overdosed America*, (New York, NY: Harper Collins, 2008)

37 Ibid.

38 https://www.publicintegrity.org/health.

39 John Abramson, *Overdosed America*, (New York, NY: Harper Collins, 2008)

40 Ibid.

41 Ibid., 96

42 Ibid., 95

43 Susannah Cahalan, "Medical studies are almost always bogus," *New York* Post, May 6, 2017. http://nypost.com/2017/05/06/medical-studies-are-almost-always-bogus/

44 John Abramson, *Overdosed America*, (New York, NY: Harper Collins, 2008)

45 Ibid.

46 Ty M. Bollinger, *The Truth About Vaccines*, Documentary, Ty M. Bollinger, 2017

47 History of Vaccine Schedule, *Vaccine Truth: Your Child, Your Choice,* https://vactruth.com/history-of-vaccine-schedule/

48 Ibid.

49 "The Childhood Immunization Schedule and Safety: Stakeholder Concerns, Scientific Evidence, and Future Studies," *The Institute of Medicine of the National Academy of Sciences,* 2013, https://www.ncbi.nlm.nih.gov/books/NBK206948/pdf/Bookshelf_NBK206948.pdf

50 Tetyana Obukhanych, Ph.D, *Vaccine Illusion: How Vaccination Compromises Our Natural Immunity and What We Can Do to Regain Our Health* (eBook, GreenMedInfo.com, 2012), 5-6

51 "The National Childhood Vaccine Injury Act of 1986," *National Vaccine Information Center,* http://www.nvic.org/injury-compensation/origihanlaw.aspx

52 "Vaccine Excipient & Media Summary, *Centers for Disease Control and Prevention,* https://www.cdc.gov/vaccines/pubs/pinkbook/downloads/appendices/b/excipient-table-2.pdf

53 "WAPF Vaccination Index," *Wise Traditions* 16, no. 2 (2015):20

54 "The ATSDR 2015 Substance Priority List," *Centers for Disease Control and Prevention,* https://www.atsdr.cdc.gov/spl/

55 Interview with Robert F. Kennedy, Jr., Ty M. Bollinger, *The Truth About Vaccines*, Documentary, Ty M. Bollinger, 2017

56 Ty M. Bollinger, *The Truth About Vaccines*, Documentary, Ty M. Bollinger, 2017

57 Ibid.

58 Ibid.

59 Neil Z Miller and Gary S Goldman, "Infant mortality rates regressed against number of vaccine doses routinely given: Is there a biochemical or synergistic toxicity?" *Human and Experimental Toxicology.* 30(9) 1420–1428, 1427

60 Neil Z Miller and Gary S Goldman, "Infant mortality rates regressed against number of vaccine doses routinely given: Is there a biochemical or synergistic toxicity?" *Human and Experimental Toxicology.* 30(9) 1420–1428

61 Ty M. Bollinger, *The Truth About Vaccines*, Documentary, Ty M. Bollinger, 2017

62 Tetyana Obukhanych, Ph.D, *Vaccine Illusion: How Vaccination Compromises Our Natural Immunity and What We Can Do to Regain Our Health* (eBook, GreenMedInfo.com, 2012)

63 Ibid.

64 Ibid.

65 Ibid., 73

66 Anthony R Mawson, Brian D Ray, Azad R Bhuiyan, and Binu Jacob, "Pilot comparative study on the health of vaccinated and unvaccinated 6- to 12- year-old U.S. children," *Journal of Translational Science,* Vol 3(3): 4-12 (2017), http://www.cmsri.org/wp-content/uploads/2017/05/MawsonStudyHealthOutcomes5.8.2017.pdf

67 Lance D. Johnson, "More children harmed by VACCINES than from GUNSHOTS, government statistics reveal," *Natural News*, May 16, 2017. http://www.naturalnews.com/2017-05-16-vaccines-are-harming-more-babies-each-day-than-gunshots.html

68 John W. Sanders and Todd A. Ponzio, "Vectored immunoprophylaxis: an emerging adjunct to traditional vaccination." *BioMed Central*, February 10, 2017, https://tdtmvjournal.biomedcentral.com/articles/10.1186/s40794-017-0046-0

69 Ty M. Bollinger, *The Truth About Vaccines*, Documentary, Ty M. Bollinger, 2017

70 Kennedy, RF, Jr., Mercury on Vaccines, *World Mercury Project*, https://worldmercuryproject.org/mercury-facts/mercury-in-vaccines/

71 Ibid.

72 Ibid.

73 Ibid.

74 Healthy People 2020, *Healthy People*, https://www.healthypeople.gov/2020/topics-objectives

75 Gates, Bill. TedTalk. February 2010. https://www.ted.com/talks/bill_gates#t-168806

Chapter 6

1 EPA TSCA Chemical Substance Inventory, https://www.epa.gov/tsca-inventory

2 "Toxic Chemicals," *Center for Responsive Politics.*, June 8, 2016, https://www.opensecrets.org/news/issues/chemical/

3 Mike Adams, *Food Forensics: The Hidden Toxins Lurking in Your Food and How You Can Avoid Them for Lifelong Health*, (Dallas, TX: BenBella Books, Inc., 2016).

4 Ibid.

5 "Fourth national report on human exposure to environmental chemcials, 2009. *U.S. Centers for Disease Control and Prevention* Updated 2017. https://www.cdc.gov/exposurereport/pdf/Fourth Report_UpdatedTables_Volume1_Jan2017.pdf and https://www.cdc.gov/exposurereport/pdf/FourthReport_UpdatedTables_Volume2_Jan2017.pdf

6   Mike Adams, *Food Forensics: The Hidden Toxins Lurking in Your Food and How You Can Avoid Them for Lifelong Health*, (Dallas, TX: BenBella Books, Inc., 2016).

7   Mark Schauss, "Toxicity and Chronic Illness," *Wise Traditions* 16, no. 1: 26.

8   Kresser, Chris. RHR: Methylation-What it is and why should you care?" *Chris Kresser*, September 11, 2014. https://chriskresser.com/methylation-what-is-it-and-why-should-you-care/

9   Ibid.

10 Mike Adams, *Food Forensics: The Hidden Toxins Lurking in Your Food and How You Can Avoid Them for Lifelong Health*, (Dallas, TX: BenBella Books, Inc., 2016).

11 Ibid.

12 Ibid.

Chapter 9

1   "Characteristics of Traditional Diets," *Weston A. Price Foundation*, https://www.westonaprice.org/health-topics/abcs-of-nutrition/principles-of-healthy-diets-2/

2   Salley Fallon Morrel and Mary G. Enig, Ph.D., *Nourishing Traditions: The Cookbook that Challenges Politically Correct Nutrition and the Diet Dictocrats, Rev. 2nd Ed.*, (Brandywine, MD: New Trends Publishing, 2001).

3   Ibid.

4   Weston A. Price, DDS. *Nutrition and Physical Degeneration*. (Lemon Grove, CA: Price-Pottenger Nutrition Foundation: 1939/2014)

5   Jordan S. Rubin, *The Maker's Diet*, (Lake Mary, FL: Siloam, 2005).

6   Salley Fallon Morrel and Mary G. Enig, Ph.D., *Nourishing Traditions: The Cookbook that Challenges Politically Correct Nutrition and the Diet Dictocrats, Rev. 2nd Ed.*, (Brandywine, MD: New Trends Publishing, 2001).

7   Ibid., 27

8   Ibid.

9   Ibid., 29

10 Sally Fallon Morell, *Nourishing Fats: Why We need Animal Fats for Health and Happiness*, (New York, NY: Grand Central Life & Style, 2017).

11 Salley Fallon Morrel and Mary G. Enig, Ph.D., *Nourishing Traditions: The Cookbook that Challenges Politically Correct Nutrition and the Diet Dictocrats, Rev. 2nd Ed.*, (Brandywine, MD: New Trends Publishing, 2001).

12 Ibid.

13 Ibid.

14 Ibid.

15 Ibid.

16 Ibid., 11

17 Ibid., 11

18 Ibid., 12

19 Kelly Brogan, M.D., "Study Links Statins to 300+ Adverse Health Effects," *Kelly Brogran*, http://kellybroganmd.com/cracking-cholesterol-myth-statins-harm-body-mind/

20 Salley Fallon Morrel and Mary G. Enig, Ph.D., *Nourishing Traditions: The Cookbook that Challenges Politically Correct Nutrition and the Diet Dictocrats, Rev. 2nd Ed.*, (Brandywine, MD: New Trends Publishing, 2001).

21 Ibid.

22 Ibid.

23 Ibid.

24 Ibid., 21

25 Ibid., 22

26 Norm Shriever, "Sweet Poison: America's deadly sugar epidemic," *Sacramento Chiropractic*, June 18, 2015, http://sacramentochiropractic.com/sweet-poison-americas-deadly-sugar-epidemic/

27 Salley Fallon Morrel and Mary G. Enig, Ph.D., *Nourishing Traditions: The Cookbook that Challenges Politically Correct Nutrition and the Diet Dictocrats, Rev. 2nd Ed.*, (Brandywine, MD: New Trends Publishing, 2001).

28 Chris Kresser, "Beyond Paleo." *Chris Kresser*, https://chriskresser.com/beyond-paleo-5/

29 Ibid.

30 Ibid.

31 "These Labels Are So Confusing!," *Grace Communications Foundation*, http://www.sustainabletable.org/944/these-labels-are-so-confusing

32 "How sweet is it?" *Harvard University*, https://cdn1.sph.harvard.edu/wp-content/uploads/sites/30/2012/10/how-sweet-is-it-color.pdf

33 Salley Fallon Morrel and Mary G. Enig, Ph.D., *Nourishing Traditions: The Cookbook that Challenges Politically Correct Nutrition and the Diet Dictocrats, Rev. 2ⁿᵈ Ed.,* (Brandywine, MD: New Trends Publishing, 2001)

34 Ibid.

Chapter 10

1   David M. Marquis, "How inflammation affects every aspect of your health," *Mercola* http://articles.mercola.com/sites/articles/archive/2013/03/07/inflammation-triggers-disease-symptoms.aspx

2   Natasha Campbell-McBride, "Healing the Body and Mind Through the Gut." ACRES. April 2016. Vol 46 No 4

3   "Global Healing Traditions." *The Herbarium*, http://herbarium.theherbalacademy.com/2016/08/advanced-herbal-course-excerpt-global-healing-traditions/

4   Chris Kresser, "Chinese Medicine Demystified (Part II): Origins of the "Energy Meridian" Myth, https://chriskresser.com/chinese-medicine-demystified-part-iii-the-energy-meridian-model-debunked/

5   Chris Kresser, "Chinese Medicine Demystified (Part III): The "Energy Meridian" Model Debunked, https://chriskresser.com/chinese-medicine-demystified-part-iii-the-energy-meridian-model-debunked/

6   Ibid.

7   Ibid.

8   Ibid.

9   Ibid.

10 Rosalee De La Foret, *Alchemy of Herbs*, (Hay House, Inc., 2017)

11 Greta Kent-Stoll, "The six tastes and Ayurvedic herbalism," *The Herbarium*, http://herbarium.theherbalacademy.com/2017/05/

the-six-tastes-and-ayurvedic-herbalism/ Accessed October 15, 2016.

12 C. Norman Shealy, *The Illustrated Encyclopedia of Healing Remedies*, (Hammersmith, London: Harper Collins Publishers, Ltd., 1998)

13 E. Richard Brown, *Rockefeller Medicine Men: Medicine and Capitalism in America*, (Lost Angeles, CA: University of California Press, 1979).

14 C. Norman Shealy, *The Illustrated Encyclopedia of Healing Remedies*, (Hammersmith, London: Harper Collins Publishers, Ltd., 1998)

15 Ibid.

16 "Homeopathic prophylaxis? Tantalizing question, surprising answer," *National Center for Homeopathy*, http://www.homeopathy center.org/homeopathy-today/homeopathic-prophylaxis-tantalizing-question-surprising-answer

Chapter 11

1 Candace B. Pert, "The Wisdom of the Receptors: Neuropeptides, the Emotions, and Bodymind," *Candace Pert*, http://candacepert. com/wp-content/uploads/2017/03/Advances-1991-Wisdom-of-the-Receptors.pdf

2 "Insufficient sleep is a public health problem," *Centers for Disease Control and Prevention*, https://www.cdc.gov/features/dssleep/index.html#References

3 Ibid.

4 Joseph Mercola, "How much sleep is "enough?" *Mercola*, http://articles.mercola.com/sites/articles/archive/2015/02/19/updated-sleep-guidelines.aspx

5 Ibid.

6 Ibid.

Chapter 12

1 Weston A. Price, DDS, *Nutrition and Physical Degeneration*. (Lemon Grove, CA: Price-Pottenger Nutrition Foundation: 1939/2014), 355

2 Natasha Campbell-McBride, "Healing the Body and Mind Through the Gut." ACRES. April 2016. Vol 46 No 4.

About The Author

Michele grew up in the country and she spent her summer days at her grandparents' house snapping beans, shelling peas, and shucking corn, while listening to her Great-Uncle Joe utter unintelligible commands to the mule pulling the plow as he tilled the soil. She loves cooking for her family and friends; it is her happy place. She is a budding herbalist, an avid reader, and loves learning.

Michele is a server by nature and she has a heart and passion for helping others. She believes that living life nourished means nourishing all aspects of life: bathing our hearts and minds in truth and in turn, nourishing our bodies with healing, wholesome foods the way God intended, as well as being intentional about self-care.

She holds a Master of Education and she is a Certified Health Coach. As an educator and a coach, Michele is passionate about guiding others into living life nourished. As a speaker, she educates on these topics. Additionally, she is certified by the Institute for Responsible Technology to speak on the reality of GMOs. As a Certified Corporate Wellness Specialist she works with companies to design and implement wellness programs.

After years of suffering from her own health issues for which conventional medicine could not provide answers, and finding solutions by addressing the foundations of health, she is dedicated to guiding you on your journey to health: body, mind, and soul.

She lives with her constant companion Sheltie dog, is mom to two remarkable adult sons, two beautiful daughters-in-love, and Nana Shell to three amazing grandchildren.

To book Michele for speaking engagements or to request additional information, go to **MicheleStanford.com.**

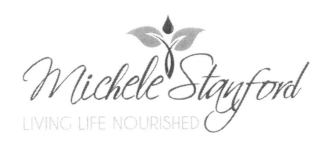

Michele Stanford

LIVING LIFE NOURISHED

It would be my pleasure and honor to serve you. I know that the information contained in *Informed Consent* has been quite a lot to take in and you're wondering where to begin. Together, we can map out your own individual journey to healing or to a healthier lifestyle for you and for your family.

I approach health from a functional, whole body perspective, meaning that health is more than just about your physical wellness. I'll ask you about your health. Your relationships. Your job. What you do for fun. What you're eating. Your spiritual life. You'll tell me what's driving you crazy. What you love. What you want to achieve. We'll determine your goals and why you want to achieve them.

We are all unique and there is no one-size fits all. My aim is to find solutions for you that fit into your all around well-being.

Let's journey together, shall we!

michele@michelestanford.com

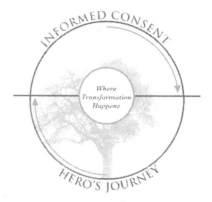

Throughout history, the archetypal hero answers the call to adventure. It may be an adventure that he needs to take to save his tribe or to save civilization. It may be an adventure to rescue a prized possession. In all of these stories from mythology to contemporary, the hero must find his courage, receive a mentor, face his enemies, and return, not only victorious, but also changed. Think of your favorite adventure stories; they all fit this profile to one degree or another.

Now it is time for you to become the hero of *your* story. In this program, I will walk with you through the 12 Stages of the archetypal hero's journey. You will recognize where you are with your health or lifestyle, discover what is holding you back, face your fear of change or resistance, either from within or from without, discover your strengths, address your health concerns or lifestyle changes with determination, and return transformed and the hero of your healing journey.

Whether you have health concerns you want to address or whether you just want to make lifestyle changes, this program is designed to help you achieve your specific, individual goals.

To begin *your* hero's journey, visit:

www.michelestanford.com/heros-journey/

Invite Michele To Your Organization

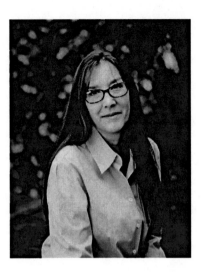

Educator – Author – Speaker – Health Coach

Michele is passionate about presenting on topics related to health and wellness. It is time to take back our pantries, food systems, personal care, food culture, and environmental choices. She invites people to get excited about that and to feel positive and motivated about nourishing themselves and their families with real, whole food, sustainably and locally produced, the way God intended.

As a speaker certified by the Institute for Responsible Technology, she loves speaking on the subject of genetically modified organisms (GMOs); their origins, the devastating health and environmental consequences.

She is happy to tailor a presentation specifically for your organization. She is passionate about sharing with others and about inviting them into living life nourished! There's so much to say!

Contact Michele to begin the conversation.

MicheleStanford.com

NOTES

NOTES

NOTES

CPSIA information can be obtained
at www.ICGtesting.com
Printed in the USA
FFOW02n0355100917
39725FF

9 781640 850439